Lesbian and Gay Nurses

Lesbian and Gay Nurses

JEFFREY ZURLINDEN, MS, RN

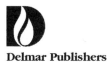

Delmar Publishers

An International Thomson Publishing Company

Albany • Bonn • Boston • Cincinnati • Detroit • London
Madrid • Melbourne • Mexico City • New York • Pacific Grove
Paris • San Francisco • Singapore • Tokyo • Toronto • Washington

NOTICE TO THE READER

Cover photo courtesy of: Spiral Design
Cover Design: Kirsten Soderlind

Delmar Staff

Senior Acquisitions Editor: Bill Burgower
Assistant Editor: Hilary Schrauf
Senior Project Editor: Judith Boyd Nelson
Production Coordinator: Barbara A. Bullock
Art and Design Coordinators: Carol D. Keohane and Timothy J. Conners

COPYRIGHT © 1997
By Delmar Publishers
a division of International Thomson Publishing Inc.

The ITP logo is a trademark under license.

Printed in the United States of America

For more information, contact:

Delmar Publishers
3 Columbia Circle, Box 15015
Albany, New York 12212-5015

International Thomson Publishing Europe
Berkshire House 168-173
High Holborn
London, WC1V 7AA
England

Thomas Nelson Australia
102 Dodds Street
South Melbourne, 3205
Victoria, Australia

Nelson Canada
1120 Birchmount Road
Scarborough, Ontario
Canada, M1K 5G4

International Thomson Editores
Campos Eliseos 385, Piso 7
Col Polanco
11560 Mexico D F Mexico

International Thomson Publishing GmbH
Konigswinterer Strasse 418
53227 Bonn
Germany

International Thomson Publishing Asia
221 Henderson Road
#05-10 Henderson Building
Singapore 0315

International Thomson Publishing—Japan
Hirakawacho Kyowa Building, 3F
2-2-1 Hirakawacho
Chiyoda-ku, Tokyo 102
Japan

1 2 3 4 5 6 7 8 9 10 XXX 02 01 00 99 98 97 96

Library of Congress Cataloging-in-Publication Data

Zurlinden, Jeffrey
    Lesbian and gay nurses / Jeffrey Zurlinden.
        p. cm.
    Includes bibliographical references and index.
    ISBN 0-8273-6970-0
    1. Gay nurses. 2. Lesbian nurses. I. Title.
    [DNLM: 1. Nurses. 2. Homosexuality 3. Interpersonal Relations.
    4. Prejudice. WY 16 Z96L 1997]
    RT82.9.Z87 1997
    610.73'06'908664 — dc20
    DNLM/DLC
    for Library of Congress   96–14482
                                                                                   CIP

DEDICATION

To the gay and lesbian nurses who because of fear and injustice remain hidden.

C O N T E N T S

Preface, xv
Acknowledgments, xxi

Chapter 1   Gay and Lesbian Lives, 1

Meaning of Lesbian and Gay, 1

Counting Gays and Lesbians, 2
The Kinsey Reports, 3
Recent Surveys, 4

Estimating Lesbian and Gay Nurses, 4

Coming Out, 5
The Six Stages, 6

Benefits of Coming Out, 10

Potential Risks, 11

Discrimination, 11

Levels of Bigotry, 12
Personal Bigotry, 12
Interpersonal Bigotry, 13
Institutional Bigotry, 15
Cultural Bigotry, 15

Why Prejudice?, 16

Stereotypes About Gay Men, 17

Stereotypes About Lesbians, 18

Summary, 20

References, 21

Chapter 2   Working with Patients, 23

Coming Out to Patients, 23

Discrimination by Patients, 24

Is Discrimination Different for Women?, 25

How Coworkers Respond, 27

Lesbian and Gay Clinics, 28

Gay and Lesbian Patients in Hospitals, 29

Patients with AIDS, 31

Steering, 32

Women Patients, 33

Working with Children, 34

Summary, 35

References, 36

Chapter 3   **Working with Coworkers and Managers, 37**

Coming Out, 37
  Why Come Out?, 38
  Personal Empowerment, 39
  Deciding Not to Come Out, 39

Methods of Coming Out, 40
  Supportive Coworkers, 41
  Coworkers Who Reject, 42
  Feeling Like an Outsider, 43

Being Outed, 46
  Dealing with Outing, 47
  Supportive Managers, 48

Using Stages of Coming Out, 49
  Stage 1: Identity Confusion, 49
  Stage 2: Identity Comparison, 49
  Stage 3: Identity Tolerance, 49
  Stage 4: Identity Acceptance, 50
  Stage 5: Identity Pride, 50
  Stage 6: Identity Synthesis, 50

Discrimination, 50
  Discrimination by Coworkers, 51
  Discrimination by Managers, 51
  Discrimination by Doctors, 53

Prejudice Based on Sectarian Beliefs, 53
  Advice from an MCC Minister, 55
  Advice from a Lesbian Christian, 56

Military Nurses, 57
  Blackmail in the Military, 57
  "Don't Ask, Don't Tell," 59

Personal Cost in the Military, 59
Fake Husbands, Fake Wives, 60

Dealing with Conflict, 60
Confronting Bigotry, 61

Working with Lesbian and Gay Nurses, 62
The Closet Community, 63

A Lesbian or Gay Boss, 63

Dating at Work, 64

Working with Your Partner, 65

Coping, 65

Summary, 66

References, 66

Chapter 4   **Legal Issues, 67**
Constant and Unpredictable Changes, 67

No Federal Protection, 68
The Federal Government as an Employer, 68

The Military, 69
Colonel Margarethe Cammermeyer, 70
Facing a Military Investigation, 72
Guidelines for Servicemembers, 72

U.S. Supreme Court, 74
Current Challenges, 75

State Protection, 76
Child Custody, 76
Sharon Kowalski and Karen Thompson, 77
State Sodomy Laws, 78
State Boards of Nursing, 78

Local Protection, 79

Protection Through Labor Contracts, 79

Summary, 81

References, 82

Chapter 5   **Domestic Partners and Benefits, 85**
No Benefits Means Discrimination, 85

Naming Committed Relationships, 86

Discrimination Against Partners, 87

How Many in Committed Relationships?, 87

Gay and Lesbian Parents, 88
    Coming Out to Children, 88
    Sharing the Responsibilities of Parenting, 89

How Relationships Grow, 90
    Gay Men, 90
    Lesbians, 91

Comparing Relationships, 92

Gay and Lesbian Relationships, 92

Sanctions for Relationships, 94

Hospitals Offering Benefits, 94
    Registering Same-Sex Domestic Partners, 95
    The University of Pennsylvania Health Systems, 95

Organizing Benefits, 95
    Collective Bargaining, 96
    Influencing Benefits without Unions, 96

The Cost of Benefits, 97

Pension Benefits, 98

Other Benefits, 98

Summary, 99

References, 99

Chapter 6   Special Problems: HIV Disease and Chemical Dependency, 101

Most Are Drug-Free and Uninfected, 102

How Many Are Infected?, 102

Nurses with HIV Disease, 103

Profiles of Nurses with HIV Disease, 103

Legal Protection, 112

ANA's Position on HIV Disease, 113

ANAC Supports Nurses, 114

Nurses Decry Mandatory Testing, 115

Advice for Nurses Infected with HIV, 116

Chemically Dependent Nurses, 117

Impaired Professional Programs, 118

Profiles of Chemically Dependent Nurses, 119

Selecting Sensitive Treatment, 126

Treatment Issues, 127

Advice for Chemically Dependent Nurses, 129

Summary, 130

References, 130

Chapter 7   Nursing Students, 133

Responsibilities to Students, 134

Coming Out, 134
    Reasons for Coming Out, 134
    Deciding Not to Come Out, 135
    Applying as an Out Student, 136
    Empowerment, 136

Student Attitudes, 137

Faculty Attitudes, 138
    Allies on Faculty, 139

Supporting Students, 140
    Stage 1: Identity Confusion, 140
    Stage 2: Identity Comparison, 140
    Stage 3: Identity Tolerance, 141
    Stage 4: Identity Acceptance, 141
    Stage 5: Identity Pride, 141
    Stage 6: Identity Synthesis, 142

Faculty Strategies, 142

Support During Clinicals, 144

Discrimination Against Students, 145
    Hate Speech and Violence, 146

Discrimination Against Faculty, 146

Cultural Competence, 147
    American Academy of Nursing Recommendations, 149
    Diversity Among Nurses, 149
    A Cultural View of Nursing School, 150
    Curriculum, 151
    Examples of Doing It Right, 152

Lesbian and Gay Role Models, 153

Find a Supportive School, 155
    Assessing Nursing Schools, 155

Surviving a Hostile Environment, 157
    Build Support, 158
    Support Groups, 159
    Survival Strategies, 159

Summary, 160

References, 162

Chapter 8   *Organized Nursing's Response, 163*

Basic Issues, 163

End Discrimination, 164
    ANA Code of Ethics, 164
    State Nurses Associations, 165
    End Discrimination in the Military, 166
    Censure Discriminatory Behavior, 166
    A National Statement, 167
    Support Coming Out, 168

Honor the History of Lesbian and Gay Nurses, 169

Ensure Culturally Competent Care, 170
    Acknowledge the Full Range of Health Issues, 171
    Use Language that Avoids Bias, 172
    Encourage Publications, 173

Support Research, 174

Benefits for Domestic Partners, 174

Employee Assistance Programs, 175

Lesbian and Gay Affinity Groups, 176
    Organizing Affinity Groups, 176
    Cassandra, 177
    The Gay Nurses' Alliance, 178

Lost Ground Due to AIDS, 179

Summary, 180

References, 180

Chapter 9   *How High the Lavender Ceiling?, 183*

Nurses Feel a Ceiling, 183

Role Models, 184
    The Lavender Network, 185

Differences Between Men and Women?, 185

Effeminate Men, Masculine Women, 186

A Generation Gap?, 187

Practice Setting, 188

Academia, 189

Interview Out?, 190
    Discrimination Is Hidden, 191

The Closet Community, 191
    Horizontal Violence, 192

The Cost of Bigotry, 194

Successful Gay and Lesbian Managers, 195

A Unique Gay and Lesbian Contribution, 196

Summary, 197

References, 198

Appendix A City of Ann Arbor, Michigan—Domestic Partnership Information Sheet, 199

Appendix B National Association of Social Workers—Policy Statement: Lesbian and Gay Issues, 203

Appendix C American Psychological Association Committee on Lesbian and Gay Concerns: Avoiding Heterosexual Bias in Language, 209

Appendix D Suggested Reading, 215

Index, 221

P R E F A C E

This book offers the opportunity to learn about the rich variety of the lives of lesbian and gay nurses. Whenever possible, I let the 108 nurses who were interviewed express their issues by quoting them directly. In doing so, I followed the advice of a nursing student who wanted to hear as many different gay and lesbian voices as possible.

This assumes that there is no right or wrong way to be lesbian or gay. Although we all have faced coming out and endured prejudice based on our sexual orientation, we make choices and live as individuals. The variety of our lives is rarely portrayed accurately by the media. Contrary to the images in glossy gay magazines, few of us are beautiful, rich, well-traveled, creative, or wildly promiscuous. Equally misleading are media images that show us as lonely, alienated, and depressed. Instead, most of us are very happily ordinary. Our lives revolve around working and maintaining relationships with our loved ones. A significant number of us are raising children. The ways that lesbian and gay nurses live in medium-sized towns in Kansas or small towns in the South are as valid and worth considering as the lives of people in New York or San Francisco.

We benefit from discussing our concerns and successes with a group of our peers. Only by hearing a broad range of points of view can we choose strategies for our own lives. Unfortunately, many gay and lesbian nurses still feel isolated because they live in small towns or more often because they fear coming out. I hope that this book feels like a living room filled with lesbian and gay nurses telling their stories.

I tried to give enough information to satisfy a general reader's curiosity, while still stimulating long-experienced gay and lesbian readers. The first chapter outlines coming out, discrimination, loving relationships, and the complex meaning of being lesbian or gay. Our work life with patients is described in Chapter 2 and with coworkers and supervisors in Chapter 3. These two chapters describe coming out at work, as well as the discrimination or support we receive as a result of that decision. The focus is on legal matters in Chapter 4 and on domestic partners in Chapter 5. Unfortunately, AIDS and chemical dependency personally affect gay and lesbian nurses, and these issues are discussed in Chapter 6. Chapter 7 describes the sometimes precarious position of nursing students, as well as the ways students are socialized to regard lesbian and gay nurses and patients. The kind of support we need and the support we get from nursing organizations is described in Chapter 8. The last chapter extends the question of coming out to include the consequences of that decision on our chances for a successful career.

To find nurses with varied experiences, I advertised in women's book stores, in *Image* (the journal of nursing's honor society Sigma Theta Tau), and in a lesbian pornography magazine. I tried to follow a standardized format, but sometimes I got engrossed in a specific issue and forgot to ask all the questions. I hope the interviews benefited from my flexibility and curiosity.

Despite my attempts to advertise in women's bookstores, gay men are overrepresented. While men account for only 4% of nurses, 37% of the nurses interviewed were men. Perhaps some women were reluctant to be interviewed by a man, or more men were willing to be interviewed by a stranger. I always tried to present women's and men's issues equally.

Many of the nurses interviewed are baby boomers. Roughly 17% are between 20 and 29 years old, 37% between 30 and 39 years, 38% between 40 and 49 years, and 7% are 50 years or older.

It is difficult to find people who are newly out and willing to talk. Luckily, 7% of the nurses interviewed were out less than 2 years, and 10% were out only 3 to 5 years. Most were out considerably longer: 19% were out 6 to 10 years, 50% between 11 and 24 years, and 15% were out 25 years or longer. "Out" meant acknowledging their gay or lesbian feelings to themselves, even if they had not yet shared their discovery with others.

Only a couple of men had children, but 30% of the women were raising either their own or their partner's children. Somewhat more, 39% of the nurses, lived with a committed partner. The length of their relationships ranged from honeymoon to over 20 years.

They have a wide range of academic backgrounds. Approximately 9% are generic nursing students, 62% have basic education, 19% have or are working on a graduate degree, and 10% have or are working on a PhD or comparable degree.

Geographically, they were well-distributed across the country in 32 states. Most live in medium-sized or suburban towns. Not surprisingly, California had the greatest number of respondents (17 nurses). It has the greatest number of women's book stores where I advertised, and a large number of nurses. Illinois was second (12 nurses), even though I tried not to concentrate in my own backyard. I interviewed nurses in the following states (the number of nurses in each state is in parentheses):

Midwest 33%	Far West 21%	East 17%
Illinois (12)	California (17)	New York (5)
Ohio (6)	Washington (4)	New Hampshire (5)
Wisconsin (6)	Oregon (2)	Pennsylvania (2)
Kansas (4)		Vermont (2)
Indiana (3)		Massachusetts (2)
Michigan (3)		Delaware (1)
Minnesota (2)		New Jersey (1)

South 15%	West 11%	Other 3%
North Carolina (4)	Texas (6)	Canada (1)
Washington, DC (2)	Colorado (3)	Alaska (1)
Virginia (2)	Nevada (2)	Hawaii (1)
Alabama (2)		
Florida (2)		
Georgia (2)		
Kentucky (1)		
South Carolina (1)		

The nurses were from all levels of nursing. Of the 108 nurses interviewed: 9% were students (10 nurses), 11% were teachers or researchers (12 nurses), 6% were directors or supervisors (6 nurses), and 11% were charge nurses or the equivalent (12 nurses).

They practiced in a wide range of clinical specialties. The 80 nurses who had clinical specialties (including charge nurses, but excluding students, teachers, and nurse managers or higher level supervisors) practiced in the following specialties: 28% ICU or high-tech (22 nurses), 19% AIDS (15 nurses), 14% psychology (11 nurses), 13% home or public health (10 nurses), 11% medical-surgical or specialty (9 nurses), 8% geriatrics (6 nurses), 5% pediatrics (4 nurses), and 5% obstetrics (3 nurses).

All of the interviews were confidential. The names used in the book are pseudonyms, but the genders remain true. In order to assure confidentiality, I sometimes omitted or changed the details of a story that could point directly to a nurse with unique circumstances. Most people were relieved that their real names would be omitted. Even out nurses found a freedom in speaking confidentially. A few nurses insisted on remaining anonymous; even I do not know their real names. Approximately 10% of the nurses questioned whether using pseudonyms gave the wrong message—that being lesbian or gay was something to be ashamed of and hide. They felt that I was pushing them back into a closet that they had struggled to leave behind.

I sympathize with their concerns. For me, being out has opened more doors than it has closed. But that is my choice, and I take the risks. I did not want anyone that helped me to be hurt as a consequence. Also, coming out has a ripple effect that may threaten the safety of the people close to us. If I used a real name, how might being out affect her partner, her children, or her best friend? Until all nurses are guaranteed not to lose their jobs, custody of their children, or risk being harassed because they are lesbian or gay, I will not feel safe using real names.

It took careful thought to decide how to handle the words *faggot* and *dyke*, which were used by many nurses without hesitation to describe encounters with bigots. These words were replaced by the words *offensive slang for lesbian (or gay man)*. All curses were deleted. Other nurses used the word *queer* to refer to all gay and lesbian people. These references were changed to *lesbian and gay* or *gay and lesbian*.

Not everyone will agree with my reasons. For me, *lesbian* and *gay* are the only words that describe us with respect, and I do not want to model disrespect. Some may argue that removing offensive words from quotations diminishes their ability to describe hatred, and others argue that removing the words imbues them with too much power.

Talking with 108 gay or lesbian nurses was invigorating. Many went way out of their way and shared intimate and perhaps dangerous information. They were willing to be interviewed out of a sense of lesbian and gay civic pride. Only one nurse called herself a bisexual, a topic that was excluded because it deserves a much longer discussion than this book could allow.

Our conversations also contained a measure of sorrow. Although most of the nurses had experienced personal growth as a result of acknowledging their gay and lesbian selves, I seldom sensed that their professional environment was once unsupportive, but now is better. Instead, it seems that individual nurses show more maturity and integrity than do nursing organizations or nursing schools; and little has changed over time.

In 1982, I put an ad in *Gay Chicago* seeking nurses to join me in the Gay Pride Parade. The only responses were friendly requests for information about the parade, solicitations for sex, and a plea to give up my sinful ways. Everyone refused to march because they might be seen on TV. By 1995, very little had changed. Although three gay and lesbian police organizations marched, the only nurses were on floats dedicated to patients— an inpatient AIDS unit, a lesbian cancer support group, and a gay and lesbian health clinic. After 12 years, the only change seems to be that it is OK for patients to be lesbian or gay, but not nurses. It is difficult to attribute nurses' reluctance to be visible entirely to a repressive political environment. There were a dozen politicians in the parade, and Chicago has an ordinance that protects gay and lesbian people. Why is the parade rolling by, while lesbian and gay nurses stand on the curb watching? As the largest minority group within nursing, why do we receive so little support from our profession? Why do we accept prejudice and neglect from our employers, professional organizations, and schools of nursing? How do these attitudes influence the care of lesbian and gay patients? Finally, how do we acknowledge and support our allies regardless of their sexual orientation?

A C K N O W L E D G M E N T S

I would like to acknowledge the encouragement of the people who listened to my sometimes half-baked ideas and helped me find the clearer path—Rosemary Camilleri, David Wallenstein, Paul Winberg, and the staff of the AIDS Research Alliance: Chicago. Special thanks are due to the reviewers Carla Randall, RN, MSN, and James Welch, RN. I apologize to the people who played phone tag with me, and I hope nurses quoted in the book also speak for you. Delmar Publishers deserves respect for having the courage to bring gay and lesbian nurses into our literature. Finally, I thank the people who sustained me—my sister Sally, Jim Lovette, Charles Straight, and José Choca who to my continuing sorrow did not live to see it completed.

1 GAY AND LESBIAN LIVES

*Being a lesbian is the most important part of my
life, yet at the same time it's not important at all.
Our lifestyle is more than just who we're attracted to.
It's just as mundane, and just as valid as anyone
else's. When you're out all the time you don't think
about it.*

A lesbian in the Midwest

MEANING OF LESBIAN AND GAY

Lesbian and gay nurses lead lives of rich variety with one com-
monality—their most genuine attraction and love is for a person
of the same gender. It is far more than a choice. Gay men and
lesbians can choose whether to acknowledge their sexual orientation and how to express it, but the roots of being lesbian or gay
are probably immutable. According to Kirsch and Weinrich
(1991), "Human homosexuality is as biologically natural as
human heterosexuality" (p. 30). Viewing sexual orientation as a
preference is offensive.

Too many people first think of gay men and lesbians in
sexual terms, as if this were the most important aspect of their
lives. Most lesbians and gay men know their sexual orientation
before they start having sex; and during periods of sexual absti-
nence, they do not stop being members of the community.

In contrast, some men and women never identify themselves as gay or lesbian and never join the community. Instead, they restrict themselves to having same-gender sex, while maintaining a heterosexual identity.

Being lesbian or gay also means forming intimate relationships with people who respect their sexual orientation. It often means loving and living with a partner of the same gender. Single gay men and lesbians usually imagine that they will one day fall in love and live with a partner. But intimate relationships show a great diversity. A sizable number of lesbians and gay men choose to live alone and draw emotional support and companionship from people who are closer than friends, or they form households with three or more members. It also means building a network of lesbian and gay companions, supporters, and friends. Unlike in some other countries, gay men and lesbians in America seldom enter heterosexual marriages in order to have children, strengthen family ties, or further their financial position.

Politically, gay men and lesbians support equal treatment of people regardless of their sexual orientation. This means establishing legal sanctions for long-term committed relationships; abandoning the barriers to child custody and adoption; and ending discrimination in employment, housing, and education. Unlike previous generations, gay and lesbian people today do not ask for tolerance or acceptance—they demand equal treatment.

This chapter lays the foundation to better understand gay and lesbian nurses and their communities. Nursing examples are used as often as possible. In the past, nursing ignored the differences between individual practitioners in order to maintain a professional—but faceless—image. Now it is time to recognize and draw strength and creativity from the diversity of individual nurses.

COUNTING GAYS AND LESBIANS

Ask any gay or lesbian person, and you will probably hear 10%; one person in ten is lesbian or gay, one nurse in ten, one auto mechanic in ten, one police officer in ten, and so on. But to researchers, the numbers depend on how you ask the question, and who asks.

Stigma may result in estimates that are too low. When asked by researchers who are strangers, some gay men and lesbians deny their sexual orientation. If same-gender sex were a felony in your state, would you answer honestly? The way the question is asked may exclude people. For example, some people who have a significant amount of sex with people of their own gender still do not think of themselves as gay, and would say "no" to the question "Are you gay?" On another survey, a woman who considers herself a lesbian could be classified a bisexual because she had sex with a man five or ten years ago. How do you classify people who do not have sex with men or women, but fantasize about people of their own gender when they masturbate?

The Kinsey Reports

Alfred Kinsey, the pioneering sex researcher, and his colleagues Wardell Pomeroy and Clyde Martin (1948/1993), graded sexual responses on a scale from 0 to 6:

0: no physical contact or emotional responses to people of their own gender that result in erotic arousal or orgasm

1: infrequent physical contact without emotional involvement that may be motivated by curiosity, while drunk, or occurred under unusual circumstances

2: more than infrequent contact, or more emotional involvement, yet their heterosexual experiences are either more frequent or emotionally meaningful

3: equal amount of physical contact and emotional involvement with men and women

4: more homosexual than heterosexual physical and emotional involvement, yet a fair amount of heterosexual activity

5: almost completely homosexual with occasional physical and emotional response to members of the opposite gender

6: all physical and emotional involvement exclusively with members of the same gender

In the 1940s, Kinsey, Pomeroy, and Martin (1948/1993) found these patterns among men: 37% had an overt homosexual experience to the point of orgasm sometime between adolescence and old age; 10% were "*more or less* exclusively homosexual" for at least three years between the ages of 16 and 55 years; 8% of men were exclusively homosexual for at least three years between the ages of 16 and 55 years; and 4% of white men were *exclusively* homosexual throughout their lives. The percentages for men of color were not reported.

Concerning women, Kinsey, Pomeroy, Martin, and Gebhard (1953/1990) found: between 11 and 20% of unmarried women and between 8 and 10% of married women had occasional lesbian experiences; and between 1 and 3% of unmarried women were exclusively lesbian.

Recent Surveys

In 1993, a large nationwide study reported that 9% of men and 5% of women admitted "ongoing" or "frequent" homosexual experiences, and 4% of men and 2% of women identified themselves as gay or lesbian (Singer & Deschamps, 1994). According to the latest "Sex in America" survey conducted by the University of Chicago, 2.8% of men and 1.4% of women identify themselves as gay or lesbian, but 10.1% of men and 8.6% of women admit to sexual experience or sexual attraction to a member of the same gender (Schirof & Wagner, 1994).

ESTIMATING LESBIAN AND GAY NURSES

No one knows how many of the roughly 2 million nurses are lesbian or gay. Because only 3 to 5% of nurses are men, lesbians far outnumber gay men. The number of male nurses is currently rising. In 1992, 11.1% of nursing students were men ("Men in Nursing," 1994). Despite the stereotype that most men in nursing are gay, men interviewed for the book complained that there are too few.

There are probably between 100,000 and 200,000 gay and lesbian nurses in America, practicing in every state, and working in every hospital and home health agency. Some are totally invisible to their coworkers, others are only known to their work friends, while a few are out to everybody. Because of stereotypes, effeminate men and masculine women are often falsely labeled as gay or lesbian.

Because there are so few members of other minority groups in nursing, lesbians and gay men are the largest minority group. According to a 1988 report, only 3.6% of RNs are Black, 1.3% Hispanic, and 2.3% Asian or Pacific Islanders ("Minorities," 1992). This means that the number of gay and lesbian nurses approximately equals all the members of racial minorities combined.

COMING OUT

Coming out means recognizing that you are gay or lesbian, and then letting other people know. Conversely, being in the closet means either refusing to recognize that you are gay or lesbian, or hiding it from others by remaining silent or ambiguous about relationships or by letting people assume you are heterosexual. Coming out is a continuum. Few people are always out; and few people, once they come out to themselves, fail to share their true identity with at least one friend or family member. The real questions of coming out are not if you will come out or when, but to whom and how.

Experienced lesbian and gay people are fluent in at least two cultures—their own, as well as mainstream heterosexual culture. Gay and lesbian people in racial or ethnic communities are fluent in additional cultures.

Unlike race, which is external, visible, and impossible to deny, sexual orientation is internal, may be invisible to a large number of people, and can be revealed selectively. Lesbian and gay people know how to pass as heterosexual when they choose to. For example, when the unknowing store clerk tells a gay man that he will make some lucky woman a fine husband, he might not say that his husband would object. Lesbians may not kiss in public if they sense it would put them in physical danger.

Coming out is a process of growth that proceeds at each person's unique pace throughout life. How fast and how far each gay and lesbian person develops depends on his or her personality, experiences, and emotional environment. Discrimination and prejudice do not promote growth.

Coming out can be described by stages that recognize the common concerns of lesbian and gay people at the same level of development. It transcends the person's age. A 20-year-old and a 40-year-old may have very different resources, competencies, and experiences; but if they have just recognized that they are gay or lesbian, they probably have very similar fears and concerns. As employees or students, they need similar support to nurture success. Describing people in a particular stage does not imply that one stage is better than another.

The Six Stages

Cass (1979) divided coming out into six stages. Examples used to illustrate each stage come from the nurses and students interviewed for this book.

Stage 1: Identity Confusion   People in this stage still see themselves as heterosexual but are plagued by a growing awareness that their feelings and behavior may be homosexual. Most people suffer this period of inner turmoil without confiding their doubts to others. One nurse recalls, "I was really asexual then. I never admitted the possibility of being a lesbian to myself because I still imagined that I would have a husband, 2.5 kids, and be the president of the PTA."

A nursing student says, "Last year I was uncomfortable going to gay and lesbian student meetings or to public gay events. I'd walk around and around the block deciding whether I'd go in, and end up going back home."

Some people cope by assuming a heterosexual identity, and a few become anti-gay and lesbian bigots in order to prove that they are heterosexuals. Others deny that they are lesbian or gay, but invent reasons why they can have same-gender sex. They might say, "I'm not gay, I just got drunk." But some people spend little time in this stage. They know they are gay or lesbian and begin exploring.

Stage 2: Identity Comparison   At this stage, people face the prospect that they might be gay or lesbian, but they do not know what it means. They are on an emotional roller coaster, uncertain how to nurture themselves, and very vulnerable. They have not yet found support from within the gay and lesbian community. They feel isolated and fear rejection.

They break through denial either in a series of small steps or in a single leap. "Suddenly there was a paradigm shift," remembers a nurse in the Midwest. "Now I see things very differently. I was terrified that people would know, because they would judge me. I didn't want people to feel any less of me. I was worried that I would be shunned and not taken seriously." As a result of the stress, she became amenorrheic, and decided to consult a new gynecologist in another town, where she could feel safely anonymous. "I was incredibly depressed. I just wasn't dealing with my lesbianism. He prescribed a drug that would return my cycle to normal. But when he asked if I was planning on becoming pregnant, I said, 'Look, I'm a lesbian.' It really shifted things for me. I thought, it's real, I said it."

Another woman remembers, "I fell in love with a woman. It hit me like a ton of bricks: I had to explore this. I wasn't certain if it was about falling in love with an individual woman, or about being a lesbian."

A staff nurse agrees, "I felt tremendous emotional turmoil and anxiety around this infatuation with a coworker. I wouldn't say anything about her for fear that my voice would betray my attraction to her. Before I fell in love, it never occurred to me that I was a lesbian. I thought it was just her."

Although people in this stage come out to themselves, they are not ready to deal with coming out to others. "I'm a very social person, but when I fell in love, I stopped eating with my coworkers. I would sit as far away as possible, and not talk much. I let them believe that I had cancer. It was more acceptable than telling the truth. All I wanted to do was be home, because there I didn't have to worry that I might blurt something out and tell the whole world that I was a lesbian."

But some people happily sail through this stage without a pause. They are relieved to have a term for who they are, and why they feel different. One nurse smiles as she says, "When I was 16 years old, I was going through an adolescent crisis, and I told my father that I thought I was a lesbian. He said, 'Your mother and I think so too.'"

Jean, who came out when she was 40 years old, found little emotional turmoil. "It happened in a natural and spontaneous way. It didn't feel like a struggle. I haven't felt blocked by any of it or been afraid by any of it. It felt wonderful. I feel more centered and grounded than I have felt during my adult life. It's a good fit."

Stage 3: Identity Tolerance   At this stage, people acknowledge that they are probably lesbian or gay, and they are very aware of the stigma. They may feel isolated, knowing that they do not fit into the heterosexual world, but not yet aware of the richness of the gay and lesbian world. Their major task is building a network of lesbian or gay friends and supporters.

One woman expresses her uncertainty: "Things that had always been the same are now different. I feel a loss of security, the personal security of a relationship, and the security of an identity, and a community. I've given up traditional ways of being a woman, but I don't yet know what I'm going to do."

They come out to other people selectively. "My first physical experience with another woman happened last summer, and I've gradually felt better and more comfortable," remembers a nursing student. "Now I feel happier and more self-confident, and I want to let the people who are close to me know about it."

Coming out to others, at this stage, often feels dangerous, intimate, and monumental. It is almost never revealed casually. The place, time, and wording may be carefully chosen and even rehearsed. At the same time, lesbians and gay men feel more genuine. If coming out was previously fraught with confusion, it now begins to make more sense. "Because I know who I am, I can better express myself, and people are more interested in knowing me. Now I can share my life with other people," says a student.

Stage 4: Identity Acceptance   At this stage, people dive into being gay or lesbian and explore the community. This is the time when they may move to San Francisco, or other areas where there are large lesbian or gay communities. Gay and lesbian cultures, or a subculture within the community, becomes the standard against which they measure behavior and relationships. They come out in a big way. Old friends and family members who respect this new identity remain close, and the others are ignored or forgotten.

Sally, an OB nurse, remembers this time well. "I finally came to the place of acceptance, and I realized that acceptance wasn't enough. I had to be proud. I felt I could be a nurse again, because you have to be present for people as a nurse. For a while, I questioned whether I could be a nurse again."

Another lesbian advises, "I'd discovered something wonderful about myself. At first, I wanted to tell the whole world, but that can get you into a lot of trouble. Don't come out to other people until you're able to take the bad punches as well as the good. It's like walking on eggshells. My feelings still get hurt. If you flaunt it in a small town, they'll all but tar and feather you."

Stage 5: Identity Pride At this stage, people feel the strongest bond to the lesbian and gay communities, political causes, and organizations. Gay men and lesbians are better than good, they are great. Many of the nurses interviewed for this book called other lesbians and gay men "family" even if they were acquaintances.

Several nurses extended themselves to provide lesbian and gay patients with extra services, attention, and kindness because they wanted to take care of "their own." Pride shows in his voice as one nurse says, "When gay people confide in you because you're gay, it's a privilege, something very special."

Nurses in this stage frequently volunteer in community organizations. "I felt that being a lesbian was so cool, so wonderful. I volunteered at a health tent at the last March on Washington, I edited the local gay newspaper. I had a rainbow flag on my locker," says a nurse from labor and delivery. Civic pride and the wish to be immersed in community also motivates some nurses to work on AIDS units.

Stage 6: Identity Synthesis People in this stage stop evaluating every issue and relationship based solely on a rigid system of lesbian or gay is good, heterosexual is suspect. Instead, they make judgments based on individual merits and potential for support, regardless of sexual orientation.

Being lesbian or gay becomes only a part, but still a vital part, of their lives. "It's difficult to explain," says a nurse who has been out for 25 years. "Being a lesbian is the most important part of my life, yet at the same time it's not important at all. Our lifestyle is more than just who we're attracted to. It's just as mundane, and just as valid as anyone else's. When you're out all the time, you don't think about it."

Their actions and beliefs express personal values. A woman who has taken many risks to express her principles as a lesbian explains, "I focus on being clear about my principles. I've learned to abandon any personal feelings of people's approval, being popular, or being in the mainstream. I focus on my purpose, why I'm doing what I do, and that what I'm doing is important."

BENEFITS OF COMING OUT

Regardless of how lesbians and gay men come out to other people, they usually feel it was worth the effort and anxiety. Almost all of the nurses interviewed for this book were out to their parents and siblings. Many were also out to at least some coworkers.

Coming out was the most common advice given by the nurses interviewed for the book. This sentiment is summarized by a nurse who has been out since she was a teenager: "All gay people owe it to themselves to be as out as possible." But why? What do you gain?

For many, coming out is eventually easier and less anxiety provoking than remaining closeted or undefined. "It took more energy not to be open about my life than to be open," says an ICU nurse.

Some nurses choose to come out directly to their coworkers because they know that they would otherwise be gossiped about. A nurse manager decided to come out to her staff because "I didn't want to be blackmailed by people who didn't get the perfect schedule."

A few nurses come out because they see it as an opportunity to promote change. "At job interviews I always ask about the hospital's policies toward domestic partners," says a gay nurse specializing in AIDS care. "I want them to know that they're discriminating against gay people by not offering benefits."

POTENTIAL RISKS

The potential benefits of coming out must be measured against the potential costs—emotional, physical, and career. As a result of discrimination, women and men have been fired from their jobs, been expelled from school, lost the support of their families, and been beaten and killed.

A successful nurse advises looking at the personal consequences of coming out, as well as the reasons for coming out. She says, "It depends on the risk-benefit ratio. If you're coming from the point of view of just venting your anger, then you shouldn't do it. If it's personally dangerous, don't do it. Rather, it should be planned to expand the number of advocates for you personally."

DISCRIMINATION

Homophobia is the word used to describe why people hate and mistreat gay men and lesbians. It explains why some people would rather hide their identity even from themselves than face the possibility that they too are a member of a hated group. By hiding, they avoid having to question the truth of this hatred. Homophobia also explains why some lesbian and gay people who are very aware of their sexual orientation may be unwilling to risk disclosing their sexual orientation.

Homophobia sounds too clinical and somehow understandable. Unmasked, homophobia is really hatred, willful ignorance, mean-spiritedness, and narrow-mindedness. It is not a psychiatric diagnosis. People suffering from homophobia do not run screaming in terror when they encounter a lesbian or gay man. Instead, they assume they are justified to be cruel; to discriminate in housing, employment, and education; and to pass laws to prevent gay men and lesbians from enjoying the civil liberties that other Americans take for granted.

Besides loving the "wrong" gender, lesbians may also be the targets of bigotry because they have intimate relationships independent of male domination. Women, regardless of their sexual orientation, risk being harassed, beaten, and killed for living strong, independent lives.

LEVELS OF BIGOTRY

Bigotry based on sexual orientation plays out, according to Warren Blumenfeld (1992), in four different levels—personal, interpersonal, institutional, and cultural. Together, these levels reinforce one another and lead to an environment that is unfriendly or hostile to lesbians and gay men.

Personal Bigotry

On the personal level, beliefs that homosexuality is bad, immoral, unnatural, or sick are better called prejudice. Many people falsely assume that nurses, because of their compassion and caring, somehow rise above the general population's prejudices. In 1991, the magazine *California Nursing* announced plans to print an article about lesbian and gay nurses. Some readers supported the article. Yet the letters to the editor also included these comments: "I am sending back the March/April issue of *California Nursing.* Please remove my name from the mailing list. I am thoroughly disgusted at the thought of receiving any literature glorifying someone's obscene sexual preferences. This is a disgrace to the nursing profession. Let's keep nursing issues on nursing—not immorality."

Another nurse wrote in part: "I was greatly disappointed to read that you are planning to publish an article on gay/lesbian RNs. By publishing such an article you will be helping to legitimize an aberrant lifestyle. As nurses, we should be concerned with public health and should not encourage behavior to spread disease. . . . "

Another wrote: "I am very offended by this article . . . . One lesbian nurse in particular is one of the best nurses I have worked with. I value her as a person and a friend, but in no way will I do anything to encourage her in the lifestyle she has chosen. As a Christian, I believe that homosexuality is a sin and represents an unhealthy, destructive lifestyle."

(The preceding letters appeared in the May/June and July/August 1991 issues of *California Nursing.* Reprinted with permission of the publisher.)

Cle Rice, the Editor in Chief, responded in an editorial preface to the article:

> . . . the responses from readers have been strong and emotional. While some nurses applauded the idea, others demanded to be taken off our mailing list at least for one issue. Still others appeared upset at the very mention of the word 'gay and lesbian nurses'—which leads us to the question: If nurses cannot acknowledge or accept gay and lesbian colleagues, how can they deliver unbiased, non-judgmental care to gay or lesbian patients or to any minority? The following article, written by award-winning writer Theresa Stephany, is in keeping with our editorial policy to give a voice to all California nurses (Stephany, 1991). (From *California Nursing*. Reprinted with permission of the publisher.)

Nurses are not alone in their negative attitudes. In June 1994, *Time* conducted a poll concerning attitudes towards gay men and lesbians to mark the 25th anniversary of New York's Stonewall Uprising, the birth of the modern gay-rights movement. In response to the question, "Are homosexual relationships between consenting adults morally wrong?" 53% said yes and 41% said no. Essentially the same responses were given to a similar survey in 1978. Although 62% of the respondents said they favored the passage of equal-rights laws to protect homosexuals against job discrimination, only 31% agreed that marriages between homosexuals should be legally recognized. Only 46% said they would allow their child to watch a TV program with a homosexual character, 42% would attend a church or synagogue with a homosexual minister or rabbi, 42% would allow their child to attend a preschool with a homosexual staff member, and only 39% said they would see a homosexual doctor. Fully 65% said that too much attention is being paid to homosexual rights (Henry, 1994).

Interpersonal Bigotry

Prejudice acted out on an interpersonal level becomes discrimination. Gay bashing, deliberately seeking lesbians or gay men to harass and injure, is the most extreme form of interpersonal bigotry. Since the federal Hate Crime Statistics Act was enacted in 1990, the FBI has collected information on crimes caused by bias. In 1991, the FBI reported that crimes against gay men, lesbians, and bisexuals accounted for 8.9% of the total 4,755 hate crimes. In 1992, the number had jumped to 11% of 8,075 crimes (National Gay and Lesbian Task Force Policy Institute, 1994). Yet many crimes go unreported to the FBI. In 1991, the National Gay and Lesbian Task Force received more than twice as many reports from just five cities—Boston, Chicago, Minneapolis and St. Paul, New York, and San Francisco—than the FBI received nationwide (Singer & Deschamps, 1994).

Because many crimes go unreported, surveys may give a clearer picture of the true extent of violence. According to a 1988 survey by the Philadelphia Lesbian and Gay Task Force, gay men, lesbians, and bisexuals are the victims of hate crimes at least four times more often than the general population. In a nationwide telephone survey, 7% of gay men, lesbians, and bisexuals said they had been assaulted at least once during the previous year because of their sexual orientation (National Gay and Lesbian Task Force Policy Institute, 1994).

How are gay men and lesbians harassed? According to a summary of 26 surveys conducted between 1977 and 1991 (Singer & Deschamps, 1994):

- ▼ 80% of victims were verbally harassed
- ▼ 44% were threatened with violence
- ▼ 33% were chased or followed
- ▼ 25% were the target of thrown objects
- ▼ 19% experienced vandalism
- ▼ 17% were physically assaulted
- ▼ 13% were spat on
- ▼ 9% were assaulted by an object or weapon

Hate crimes frequently go unreported because the police are viewed as part of the problem. They may refuse to take the report, accuse the victim of inciting the crime, or are themselves the perpetrators. In 1993 in Chicago, lesbians and gay men complained of 29 acts of police misconduct, including verbal abuse, physical abuse, sexual abuse, false arrests, and refusal to take a report (Horizons, 1994).

One nurse reported that after she came out in a small town, the word *lesbian* was spray painted on the back of her house.

Her house was also egged, and she received hate mail and phone calls.

Institutional Bigotry

Institutional bigotry can be more insidious, damaging, and difficult to change than interpersonal bigotry. Institutions are hospitals, schools, government, churches, nursing organizations, or insurance companies. Employers discriminate through hiring, promotion, and disciplinary practices that systematically work against lesbians and gay men. Sometimes the policy is written and acknowledged. For example, the military openly discriminates against gay and lesbian nurses. Civilian employers discriminate when they deny insurance or pension benefits to same-sex domestic partners.

The policy to discriminate does not have to be official to be in effect. One former nursing instructor, who remained closeted during her tenure, remembers that the admissions counselors would call when they had a presumed gay man applying to nursing school and say, "This guy is pretty effeminate, I'm sure you don't want him." If this incident involved a single counselor, who was acting out of personal prejudice, it would have been an example of interpersonal discrimination. Because the same message was delivered by many counselors, it represented a tacit institutional policy to discriminate.

Cultural Bigotry

Cultural bigotry represents the views of an entire society or culture. It is expressed first by a conspiracy of silence. Why are gay and lesbian people so seldom portrayed on television or in movies, and when they are portrayed, why are they either portrayed as buffoons or killed off? Why have lesbian and gay organizations had to go to court in order to be listed in the yellow pages? Why do official reports grossly underestimate the number of demonstrators at gay and lesbian civil rights rallies? Why do heterosexuals know so little about lesbian and gay people?

The reason is rooted in power and control. Making gay and lesbian people invisible or undercounted diminishes their political clout. They become unworthy of the services and civil rights protections that others take for granted. Lesbian and gay work-ers are easier to discipline if they fear losing their jobs, and they are cheaper to employ when benefits are withheld from their partners.

Professional literature can also be an instrument of cultural bigotry. For example, two articles in the Fall 1992 issue of the *Journal of Christian Nursing* entitled "Leaving the Lesbian Lifestyle" and "Can Homosexuals Really Change?" ignored 30 years of professional research by presenting a biased message that invalidates lesbian and gay people (Young, 1992; Moberly, 1992).

Anti-lesbian and gay bias also masquerades as fact in secular journals. Dr. Sandra Schwanberg (1990), a nurse, looked at all articles mentioning gay men and lesbians in the nursing, medical, and psychological literature from 1983 to 1987. Each of 59 articles was classified as presenting a positive, neutral, or negative image. Positive images portrayed being lesbian or gay as a "normal life-style or a variation of human behavior." Negative images said that "homosexuality was a perversion, evidence of mental illness, a stigmatized condition, or some other problem." By comparing her results with an earlier study from 1974 to 1983, she looked for changes in the image of lesbian and gay people resulting from the AIDS epidemic. There were more negative comments (36 out of 59) in the newer publications. But nursing literature had more positive or neutral images than either medicine or psychiatry. Out of 17 total nursing articles, 7 were negative, 4 were positive, and 6 were neutral.

Labeling gay and lesbian civil rights as "special rights" is another form of cultural bigotry. This cultural bigotry is best carried out by an environment that makes coming out dangerous.

WHY PREJUDICE?

Americans voice a wide range of opinions about gay and lesbian people, from fervent support to outright hostility. Dr. Gregory Herek (1992), a social psychologist and an expert on anti-lesbian and gay violence, answered why some people are prejudiced. What function does the person's attitudes serve? Some people are strongly influenced by one of the following functions, and others are influenced by a combination of the following functions.

▾ **Experience:** Past experience with gay and lesbian people guides a person's future opinions and actions. People who have had positive experiences develop generally positive attitudes. But less than 25% of the people Dr. Herek studied were influenced by experience.

▾ **Self-expression:** Over 40% of the people studied based their attitudes on strongly held personal values, or the opinions of others who were important to them. For example, some religious sectarians may condemn gay and lesbian lifestyles because the condemnation confirms their beliefs of themselves. Bigotry is an expression of their values. Or, some people ridicule lesbian and gay people as a way to win the admiration of people who they assume share these attitudes. Bigotry is a tool for social success.

▾ **Defense:** About 25% of the people studied used negative attitudes as a way to reduce their anxiety. Conflicts or confusion about their own sexuality or gender led them to condemn lesbians and gay men, rather than deal with their own risky desires.

STEREOTYPES ABOUT GAY MEN

Negative stereotypes are another manifestation of cultural bigotry that deny that gay men and lesbians are individuals. Stereotypes about gay men include:

Molest Children A recent article in the prestigious journal *Pediatric* reviewed 269 confirmed cases of sexual abuse and found only two offenders who were lesbian or gay. Children are usually sexually abused by heterosexual members of their close family or family friends. Fully 82% of the offenders were in this category. The most common offenders were fathers (40.2% for female victims and 36% for male victims), mothers' boyfriends (11.9% for female victims and 16% for male victims), and step-fathers (11.4% for female victims and 6% for male victims) (Jenny, Roesler, & Poyer, 1994).

Hate Women   Almost all of the men interviewed for the book maintained close friendships with at least one woman.

Effeminate, Really Want to Be Women   Effeminacy is a separate characteristic: some gay men are effeminate, some heterosexual men are effeminate.

You Can Tell a Bird By Its Feathers   This myth is perpetuated by the stand-up comedian's portrayal of limp-wristed, lisping, mincing homosexual characters that are no more true than step-'n-fetch-it images of African Americans. There is a rich diversity among gay men in appearance, character, and behavior.

All Gay Men Have AIDS   Researchers cannot accurately estimate the number of gay men who are infected with HIV. Even in cities at the heart of the epidemic, fewer than half of gay men are infected.

Sensitive and Caring   Although many gay men in nursing are proud that they can tune into their patients' needs, it is a skill they developed. Gay men have a full range of feelings and needs. It is unreasonable to expect gay men to always silently shoulder the burden of being sensitive and caring.

Entertaining, Witty, and Urbane   This belief trivializes the opinions of gay men. As one nurse puts it, "Gay men are the ones who are supposed to make the really fabulous spinach dip and sing Cole Porter tunes. But not make any of the big decisions."

STEREOTYPES ABOUT LESBIANS

Researchers (Eliason, Donelan, & Randall, 1992) surveyed nursing students to uncover common stereotypes about lesbians. Fourteen percent of the students felt that lesbians are "biologically unnatural," and 13% objected to lesbians for "moral, ethical, or religious" reasons. The students showed five recurrent themes (the comments that follow each section are from the author):

Lesbians Seduce Heterosexual Women   Over one-third of the nursing students indicated that heterosexual women are frequently the target of lesbian sexual advances. "Respondents suggested 'keeping a distance' from all lesbians to 'protect' themselves from those 'overly friendly' lesbians who will 'make eyes at you' or 'put the moves on you.'" Because most of the students were between 19 and 22 years old, these comments may reflect sexual inexperience, as well as youth's preoccupation with sex.

Comments: One of the students interviewed for this book said that after she overheard comments from her nursing classmates about lesbian temptresses, she was more reluctant to come out at school. She also says, "With all the interesting and eligible lesbians out there, why would I waste my time seducing narrow-minded straight girls?"

Lesbians Want to Be Men   Just under one-third of the nursing students thought that you could spot a lesbian by the mannish way she dresses, cuts her hair, and avoids makeup. Along with this, lesbians are also presumed to be good at sports, know how to use power tools, and generally act like men.

Comments: Over half of the lesbian nurses interviewed for this book said that strangers would be unable to identify them as lesbians because they use makeup, wear dresses at socially appropriate times, and have long hair.

A Chicago nurse also told the following joke: "There's this stereotype that all lesbians drive pickup trucks. But it's not true—there are not nearly enough pickup trucks." She also lamented after a vacation in the Pacific Northwest, "It was very frustrating. The place is filled with healthy looking women, without makeup, wearing flannel shirts—and almost all of them are straight."

A related aspect of this stereotype says that lesbians hate men. Over half of the nurses interviewed for this book were married at one point, and almost all count men among their friends and social companions.

The positive side of this stereotype portrays lesbians as competent because they are perceived to approximate men. In contrast, gay men are incompetent because stereotypically they approximate women.

Lesbians Are Too Blatant   Twenty-nine percent of the students felt that lesbians tried to push their lifestyle on heterosexuals. Said one student, "I would hope that this type of woman would respect me and others and not talk about her life-style freely." Another said, "They are not normal human beings. They try to turn young, normal people into lesbians with their gay marches."

Comments: Ironically, the most common method of coming out at work among the lesbians interviewed for this book was to talk about their lives in the same way that heterosexual women talk about theirs. For example, when the discussion is about marriage, lesbians talk about their partners. They considered this style low-key and not offensive.

Lesbians Are a Bad Influence on Children   Fewer students, 11%, responded that lesbians were poor role models for children, although only three students mentioned sexual molestation.

Comments: The high number of lesbian mothers and the almost nonexistence of lesbians who sexually abuse children suggests that children are safe and well-nurtured by lesbians.

Lesbians Spread Sexually Transmitted Diseases   Twenty-eight percent of the students agreed with the statement, "Lesbians are a high risk group for AIDS," and 13% wrote about AIDS in open-ended questions.

Comments: It is disappointing that so many students failed to understand how HIV is transmitted. Women who have sex exclusively with women are much less likely than heterosexual women to become infected with HIV. However, women, regardless of their sexual orientation, are at risk if they share needles during injection drug use. This may reflect a more pervasive stereotype that labels outcasts as "unhealthy."

SUMMARY

Lesbians and gay men participate in a network of interconnected subcultures that together form a rich and varied community. All gay men and lesbians have dealt with the issues of admitting their sexual orientation to themselves, as well as how and when to disclose to others. They have all had to reevaluate the tenets of mainstream, heterosexual society in terms of their own sexual orientation, and conclude that for them being lesbian or gay is genuine, immutable, and good.

Discrimination and the unequal distribution of rights and benefits still exists. Many gay men and lesbians today still live in a world no less bigoted than was Montgomery, Alabama, before Dr. Martin Luther King led the bus boycotts in the 1950s. Examples in the following chapters strongly illustrate how the issues of coming out and discrimination influence lesbian and gay nurses. Some examples show the needless waste of discrimination, and others show how supervisors, coworkers, instructors, and organizations can support gay and lesbian nurses so that coming out can be a personal decision unfettered by the fear of retribution.

References

Blumenfeld, W. (Ed.). (1992). *Homophobia: How we all pay the price.* Boston: Beacon Press.

Cass, V. C. (1979). Homosexual identity formation: A theoretical model. *Journal of Homosexuality, 4*(3), 219–235.

Eliason, M., Donelan, C., & Randall, C. (1992). Lesbian stereotypes. *Health Care for Women International, 13*(2), 131–144.

Henry, W. (1994, June 17). Pride and prejudice. *Time, 143*(26), 57–59.

Herek, G. M. (1992). Stigma, prejudice, and violence against lesbians and gay men. In J. Gonsiorek & J. Weinrich (Eds.), *Homosexuality: Research implications for public policy* (pp. 60–80). Newbury Park, CA: Sage.

Horizons. (1994). *Chicago anti-violence project statistics 1993.* Chicago: Horizons Community Services.

Jenny, C., Roesler, T. A., & Poyer, K. L. (1994). Are children at risk for sexual abuse by homosexuals? *Pediatrics, 94*(1), 41–44.

Kinsey, A., Pomeroy, W., & Martin, C. (1993). Sexual behavior in the human male. In W. B. Rubenstein (Ed.), *Lesbians, gay men, and the law* (pp. 1–12). New York: The New Press. (Original work published 1948)

Kinsey, A., Pomeroy, W., Martin, C., & Gebhard, P. (1990). Sexual behavior in the human female. In W. B. Rubenstein (Ed.). *Lesbians, gay men, and the law* (pp. 12–15). New York: The New Press. (Original work published 1953)

Kirsch, J. A., & Weinrich, J. D. (1991). Homosexuality, nature, and biology: Is homosexuality natural? Does it matter? In J. C. Gonsiorek and J. D. Weinrich (Eds.), *Homosexuality: Research implications for public policy* (pp. 13–31). Newbury Park, CA: Sage.

Men in nursing: How the ranks are growing. (1994). *RN, 57*(2), 14.

Minorities: Still not many in nursing. (1992). *RN, 55*(4), 12.

Moberly, E. (1992). Can homosexuals really change? *Journal of Christian Nursing, 9*(4), 14–17.

National Gay and Lesbian Task Force Policy Institute. (1994). Anti-gay/lesbian/bisexual violence fact sheet. Washington, DC: National Gay and Lesbian Task Force.

Schirof, J., & Wagner, B. (1994, October 17). Sex in America. *U.S. News & World Report, 117,* 74–81.

Schwanberg, S. L. (1990). Attitudes towards homosexuality in American health care literature 1983–1987. *Journal of Homosexuality, 19*(3), 117–136.

Singer, B., & Deschamps, D. (Eds.). (1994). *Gay and lesbian stats: A pocket guide of facts and figures.* New York: The New Press.

Stephany, T. M. (1991). The invisible presence: Gay and lesbian nurses. *California Nursing, 13*(3), 20–22.

Young, M. (1992). Leaving the lesbian lifestyle. *Journal of Christian Nursing, 9*(4), 10–13.

Chapter

2 | WORKING WITH PATIENTS

*People in the hospital put their trust in a stranger,
and that stranger is you. It's an honor that you
haven't earned as a person, but because you are a
nurse, and people trust nurses. So you have to treat
all clients well regardless of their sexual orientation,
or any other personal thing about them.*

A lesbian nurse

COMING OUT TO PATIENTS

Nurses describe different strategies for coming out. Some decide to keep their sexual orientation entirely to themselves. "My patients don't know anything about my personal life. It's my policy." Another says, "I maintain a professional demeanor with my patients, and focus on them." A new grad says, "I will never come out to a patient while they're still a patient. At discharge, if we have a bond, I'll tell."

Others let the patients determine how much they want to know. "If they ask me directly, I answer truthfully. I think that most of them assume that I'm gay, but I don't make an issue of it. I don't broadcast it." Some nurses take cues from the patient in terms of intimacy. If the relationship remains superficial, the nurse does not come out. But if the patient discloses intimate information, she considers coming out.

23

Many nurses reiterated that their relationship with the patient is a therapeutic one based on the patient's needs. As an out lesbian in Florida explains, "When I feel the urge to divulge personal information, I first step back and see if it benefits me, or benefits my patients. Usually it doesn't benefit them, so I don't talk about my personal life."

At times, unusual situations arise. A San Francisco lesbian recalls, "If an older person asks if I'm married, I say yes and don't pursue it. But one time an old woman said to me, 'I have a stupid question. Are you a boy or a girl?'"

Although he usually does not disclose his sexual orientation to patients, a medical-surgical nurse admitted to being gay when a woman asked him directly. But she prefaced her question with the comment, "No male nurse, other than a gay man, could be as caring and compassionate as you are."

Unfortunately, some nurses remain closeted at work because of fear of patient reactions. A young gay staff nurse describes his concerns: "The hardest thing we go through is that we have this gay culture that embraces us in every way. But when you go to work, you have to leave it at the door. If I were openly gay at work, the patients would refuse to let me care for them or demand to know my HIV status."

DISCRIMINATION BY PATIENTS

Cruel, vicious statements by patients are almost always unexpected. "I was shocked," remembers a gay pediatric nurse. "A teenage girl suddenly screamed (*offensive slang for gay man*) at me. I used my dad voice to tell her that I was an adult, and I expected to be treated with respect. I also told her that I let most children call me by my first name, but that it was a privilege, and from now on, she could only refer to me as Mr. ___."

Gay-bashing remarks by patients also hurt nurses who are not out. A lesbian from a small town, "just a dot on the map," who was struggling with coming out remembers caring for a bigoted man:

> He pointed to an effeminate orderly and told me, "You can smell them (*offensive slang for gay men*) a mile away, they

should be shot." It tore me apart that he could be so biased. It made me mad. I decided you can't trust people, even when you think you know them. Rejection would have cut me deep. I had to keep my distance when he wanted to be personal. I avoided caring for him. He thought he knew me, but he didn't know me at all.

Ted Felt Wounded

Discrimination can also be disguised by a calm voice. Ted describes a middle-aged woman who refused to let him care for her on an ICU. When he asked why, she replied, "Don't make me say it. You know what you are."

"It was humiliating," he explains. "I felt wounded, discriminated against, but more subtly because she used a soft voice and was alert." His solution was to switch assignments with another nurse, but it exacted an emotional cost. "Changing the assignment had its own peculiar sadness. It was yet another example of the relentless force of bigotry."

Ted could have tolerated the situation easier if the patient had been loud and belligerent. Because she seemed otherwise reasonable and intelligent, it forced him to focus on the content of her prejudice.

IS DISCRIMINATION DIFFERENT FOR WOMEN?

Many lesbians said that they were not the targets of discrimination because they more easily pass as heterosexuals in a patient's eyes. Many echoed the sentiments of a medical-surgical nurse in the Midwest who says, "Unless I looked my patients right in the eye and screamed, 'I am lesbian,' they would never catch on."

Yet, despite their seeming invisibility, several lesbian nurses reported being the target of a patient or family member's bigotry. One nurse recalls when her patient's son announced at the nurse's desk, "Don't let that (*offensive slang for lesbian*) do CPR on my mother."

A nurse describes an incident that happened to a lesbian colleague who practices in a small town. While the nurse was changing a woman's hysterectomy dressing, the patient asked if she was a lesbian. When she answered truthfully, "The patient went ballistic and said, 'Get out of my room, you've seen me spread-eagled.'"

Bette Confronts Prejudice

Bette is an out lesbian and a home health nurse in the rural West. She describes an incident involving a patient's mother who complained about Bette to the home health aide, rather than criticizing Bette directly. Bette explains: "The aide felt that I was entitled to know what was being said about me behind my back. The mother said very hurtful, hateful things, including that I frequented a lesbian cathouse, and that she couldn't trust me alone with her daughter."

But Bette felt that the aide was supportive. "She let me know the comments were inappropriate because in her eyes my being a lesbian didn't affect the care the patient received."

She dealt with the problem by confronting the patient's mother directly. "I told her that if she had a problem with the care I was providing, then it was important to report me to my boss, rather than talking with the aide."

The mother never reported her and stopped gossiping about her as well. The strategy worked because Bette delivered excellent nursing care and was respected for it. She was out to her boss since the time of their initial interview. She did not have to worry about losing her job just because she was a lesbian. Being out helped to focus the issue where it belonged: on the quality of nursing care.

HOW COWORKERS RESPOND

The drama of discrimination may play out behind closed doors in the relative isolation of a patient's room or in front of a full audience in the hospital's corridors or in an ICU fishbowl. Wherever the incident occurs, gay and lesbian nurses complain that few coworkers offer their support.

One man tells of an instance when he taught a pre-operative preparation class for children scheduled for elective surgery. On the evaluation form, a parent wrote, "Don't let the (*offensive slang for gay man*) nurse near any more children." The comment did not hurt as much as the silence that followed. He explains: "Even though my supervisor read every evaluation form, she never told me that the parent's comment was wrong, and that she valued my contribution. Her silence seemed to say that she agreed with the comment."

Another man describes a public display in a neurology ICU by a psychotic and paralyzed teenager. "He was making fun of me in a mocking effeminate voice and screamed (*offensive slang for gay man*) at me," he explains. "I was embarrassed. My coworkers just ignored it, but didn't support me. If I had been more out, I think the staff would have been more supportive. You have to give them an opportunity to support you."

There may be more support in hospitals that attract a larger number of openly lesbian and gay nurses. A gay man working as a shift supervisor in such a hospital remembers, "We were in a meeting about harassment when a supervisor brought up an instance when a patient screamed (*offensive slang for gay man*) at a gay male nurse. Her response was supportive. She said that he was an excellent nurse, and the remarks were uncalled for. She didn't try to blame the victim."

Burt Expected Support

Burt is out. He intentionally chose to work in a hospital with a policy against discrimination on the basis of sexual orientation. He also made it clear that he expected his supervisor to support him. He explains: "I was teamed with a new grad. One of our patients was a middle-aged man who needed to have a urinary catheter removed. First he told the new grad to get lost, then he asked me if I was gay. I asked him why he wanted to know, but he kept arguing. I left and called patient relations and my manager."

Because the nurses were unionized, the manager's response was clear. According to Burt, "The manager told patient relations and the patient that the hospital has a policy of nondiscrimination, and that she couldn't guarantee that the nurse wouldn't be gay, white, black, a man, or a woman. Later he apologized on his own, and we didn't have any more problems."

The manager's support did not stem from friendship. Instead, she supported Burt because she knew he would file a grievance if she failed to support him. His advice to lesbian and gay nurses, "Don't appear like a target. Managers frequently see gay and lesbian people as more vulnerable. Don't be arrogant, but don't be weak or soft, or you will become a victim. Defend yourself, join the union, file grievances."

LESBIAN AND GAY CLINICS

Many lesbian and gay nurses fantasize about working in an environment free of bigotry and harassment, where they can openly talk about their lovers, where their sexual orientation is valued and respected, and where they can help other gay and lesbian people. In short, they dream about working in a gay and lesbian health clinic.

A man who worked at a lesbian and gay clinic for three years explains why he wanted to work in the clinic: "I always wanted to know what it would feel like not to have to wonder if I was being criticized just because I'm a man, because I'm gay, or because of what I do. Working in a gay clinic helped me work that out."

Another nurse says, "I grew up a lot. I came with a certain amount of rebelliousness. I wanted to be outrageously gay and do everything I could never get away with in a hospital. But as time went on, I learned to focus on the patient and not to let my style be the center of attention. Without being forced to behave in a certain way, I discovered that I'm not very outrageous. I became confidently gay and a nurse."

Other nurses stop looking at the lesbian and gay world through rose-colored glasses after working in a gay clinic. "Whoever said that gay men are sensitive and caring never worked here. I found out that gay people are like anyone else. I worked with some good people, but also people who didn't have a clue how to support you or work as a team. They were too busy flirting or gossiping."

Lesbian and gay communities have some of the same drawbacks as the smallest of small towns. A lesbian comments, "Working in a gay clinic blurs the boundaries between personal and professional life. Clients would come in and complain because they overheard a staff person in a bar talking about things they shouldn't be talking about."

For many, the closeness eventually became too much. According to a gay nurse who left on good terms, "The secrets I knew about clients felt like burdens. I left the clinic because I needed a little more distance from work."

GAY AND LESBIAN PATIENTS IN HOSPITALS

Lesbian and gay patients usually sense that hospitals are hostile places and act guarded. A lesbian nurse explains:

> I could tell that the patient was a lesbian and the other woman was her lover, but they seemed uncomfortable in a distant way. So I asked, "Are those matching rings? My lover and I have matching rings too." Then they seemed more comfortable touching and supporting each other in the hospital, and they were friendlier with me.

Another nurse describes an openness shared by a gay nurse and gay patient, "There are times when the patients don't tell the doctor because they're more comfortable talking with someone who they assume is gay." Part of the issue might be cultural competence. Does the doctor know how to ask questions in a gay or lesbian-sensitive fashion? Or does the patient feel that risking disclosing a lesbian or gay identity to the doctor or other heterosexual staff might result in poor treatment or ridicule?

Some nurses risk the stigma of coming out by caring for lesbian and gay patients. A nurse in a rural area now volunteers to care for gay and lesbian patients because, "they're very vulnerable, and they need support. It's a bond and acknowledging it is to both our benefits. In the past, I was afraid to care for a lesbian patient because it would have tipped people off that I was gay."

A nurse in California remembers when a patient came up to the nurse's station wearing a t-shirt with the printed message, "1 in 10: It's a gay thing, you wouldn't understand." A heterosexual nurse read the shirt and admitted that she did not understand. "I said, 'Of course you wouldn't.' Both the patient and I cracked up. He almost wet his pants. He knew he had a friend on the unit."

Most lesbian and gay patients are hospitalized for health problems unrelated to AIDS, and may be admitted to any hospital unit. For example, an ICU nurse says, "I had to advocate to allow the significant other to visit when her lover was dying. The staff was then supportive."

Nurses on psychiatric units said they come out to gay or lesbian patients if it helps develop rapport and enables the patient to more easily explore his or her issues. Sometimes the nurse almost acts as a role model of an emotionally healthy lesbian or gay person.

Other nurses describe acting as teachers or liaisons for lesbian and gay patients to the staff. Nurses who are out to their coworkers are frequently respected for their specialized expertise. They welcome the opportunity to care for gay and lesbian patients.

A child psychiatric nurse describes the lack of expertise in psychiatry in dealing with patients who are gay or lesbian, "They either don't want to deal with it, or overemphasize the gayness to explain the whole problem." He offers his expertise and makes referrals to resources within the lesbian and gay communities.

PATIENTS WITH AIDS

Many nurses described heroic efforts to ensure that patients with AIDS got sensitive and humane care. "With AIDS patients we show more compassion, because it hits home, it's a family problem," says a nurse who otherwise does not come out at work because she does not trust her coworkers to help her if she did.

Another nurse who was very afraid to come out at work, because the "administration would find some reason to get rid of me," risked coming out to a patient with AIDS. "I asked about his partner, and we talked about mine. I'd like to think it was easier for him to be cared for by someone who didn't blame him and wasn't very moralistic about AIDS."

A nurse from the Midwest says:

> What pushed me out of the closet was the AIDS epidemic. My coworkers were so homophobic in front of patients. It was really ugly. The fear and disgust about gay people reveals a spiritual void in straight people, which if it were expressed in a way that wasn't socially sanctioned would be recognized as a psychiatric disorder. We would insist that they get professional help.

Another woman recalls:

> At first there was a lot of discrimination against gay men with AIDS. So I volunteered to care for them. My coworkers said, "Why do you like taking care of (*offensive slang for gay men*) so much?" "Because he's a human being, and the way he loves doesn't matter," I answered. In my book, it's not OK to leave people who are dying alone in a room to die. Nurses are so ignorant about how HIV is spread and how to use universal precautions. They wear space suits to care for a presumed gay man, but won't even wear gloves to care for a cute grandma who was infected with HIV during bypass surgery.

Besides being patient advocates, lesbian and gay nurses act as teachers to correct common misconceptions about HIV disease and how it is spread. By word and example gay and lesbian nurses are probably responsible for more training about AIDS and universal precautions than all the OSHA-mandated in-service classes combined.

When the full story of AIDS is told, lesbian and gay nurses will be among the heroes: working on AIDS units when few others were willing to take the risk; volunteering outside of work to care for sick and dying friends and lovers; answering seemingly endless questions regardless of the time of day; risking harassment and discrimination at work to advocate for patients with AIDS; speaking about AIDS at schools, churches, and other organizations; influencing nursing organizations, hospitals, and public health systems to address AIDS; and sometimes going public with their HIV disease, when they thought it would make a difference.

For lesbian and gay nurses, caring for people with AIDS expresses the strongest feelings of pride, compassion, and community. A lesbian in San Francisco says, "It can't be over-emphasized the amount of energy committed to AIDS by the lesbian community. AIDS has galvanized the community. This is where the heart is. I feel such a passion for my work, and that passion has sustained me."

STEERING

Few nurses reported being steered away from a practice specialty solely on the basis of their sexual orientation. However, one nurse remembers, "In the Navy, I was under investigation to try to bust my friends. After I came out, they tried to prevent me from working on peds."

Pediatric and OB nurses usually think twice before they come out to their coworkers for fear of having to deal with the unfounded stereotype of lesbians and gay men as child molesters, seducers, or recruiters into the lifestyle. An OB nurse recalls, "I decided that as a lesbian who is touching women's labia in OB, it could be wrongly assumed that I'm touching women for sexual excitement. That I should be cautious about who I tell I'm a lesbian."

Several men complained of differences in assignments based on gender. Says one staff nurse, "Because you're a man, you get the 350-pound patient who's incontinent of stool." Other openly gay men complained that they might be assigned all the AIDS patients on the floor regardless of their acuity, and they would be expected to care for them without help.

Legal decisions have been inconsistent regarding the legality of steering based on gender. A California Fair Employment and Housing Commission recently agreed with a hospital's ban against men nurses in labor and delivery because they would see female patients nude and do vaginal exams (Ban, 1994). However, in another case, the Ohio Supreme Court ruled that a nursing home could not refuse to hire men as nurses' aides out of concern for female patients' privacy (Males, 1992). It is taken for granted that male patients have no say in the gender of their nurses.

Regardless of their specialty, some lesbians are attracted to nursing because most of their coworkers are women. Says one woman who has practiced in a variety of specialties, "I knew that I preferred to socialize with women, and nursing was a perfect way to do that. I knew that I would be working with bright women."

Many nurses who work on dedicated AIDS units do so as an expression of their lesbian and gay civic duty. Explains one AIDS nurse, "I choose AIDS care out of a desire to do something for my own community. Coming out of religious life, I also need to practice in a way that fulfills a sense of social justice." Choosing to care for other gay or lesbian people also has an aspect of nurturing oneself.

WOMEN PATIENTS

For some lesbians, nurturing other women is a way of also nurturing and honoring themselves. A nurse in labor and delivery says, "When I was coming out, it was important to be woman-centered. Helping women in labor let me know that I was helping women." She remained closeted partly out of fear that her motives might be misunderstood.

Several nurses developed strategies to prevent false accusations of sexual harassment involving female patients. A lesbian nurse practitioner insists on having a chaperon in the room when she examines a woman. "I don't want a husband going off and screaming that a lesbian touched his wife. A chaperon verifies that the patient is safe. I also don't want anyone saying, 'Look how long she's taking to do a breast exam.'"

WORKING WITH CHILDREN

Pediatric units present dilemmas for lesbian and gay nurses. The atmosphere on the unit is usually informal, and pediatric nurses usually reveal and give more of their personal selves to enable families to feel safe. But stereotypes falsely paint gay and lesbian people as untrustworthy with children. "It's a unique situation; we still suffer from these archaic attitudes about gay people concerning children," says a pediatric nurse.

Marty Loses a Friend

Marty, a pediatric nurse, was hurt after she came out to an adolescent patient with a terminal illness. "He was a really cool kid; and because he was in the hospital so much, we became friends. He even met one of the women I dated."

As their friendship grew, Marty became more relaxed about answering his questions. She knew that exploring intimacy in relationships is a developmental milestone of adolescence, and she reasoned that he was vicariously exploring through his questions. Because of his illness, he would have few other opportunities to learn about relationships. When he asked about her relationships with women, she answered truthfully.

She assumed that her friendship was beneficial for the boy. She says, "His parents knew, and I didn't think there was a problem until I called his mom to ask about going to the funeral. She cursed and said, 'I never want to talk to you again. You told my son exactly how lesbians have sex.'"

As Marty told the story, she started to cry. "It caused me incredible pain to know that I might have hurt someone. My coworkers were very supportive. I cried and cried. I'll challenge homophobic or racist comments. But people are very protective about their kids. So now I use gender nonspecific terms to talk about my dates."

SUMMARY

Most lesbian and gay nurses only come out to patients after careful consideration of whether their disclosure will help the patient. They are more likely to come out to gay and lesbian patients, because it reduces the patient's sense of isolation. Most hospitals are hostile places for lesbian and gay patients, and they need a culturally competent advocate.

Although some gay and lesbian nurses avoid caring for lesbian and gay patients because they fear discrimination from their coworkers, the AIDS epidemic and the prejudicial responses by many nurses have forced some gay and lesbian nurses to risk coming out to ensure humane care for patients. Lesbian and gay nurses shoulder a disproportionate share of the responsibility of caring for people with AIDS. This commitment reflects their deep pride in their communities.

Discrimination by patients continues. Sometimes coworkers support their lesbian and gay colleagues, but too often incidents are ignored, giving the impression that the bystanders silently agree with the discrimination. Nurses who are out to their coworkers and supervisors get more support and deal with patient discrimination easier.

A lesbian who practices on an AIDS unit in a community hospital argues when she is forced to float. Part of her complaint centers on inequity: she is expected to float off the AIDS unit, while nurses from other units are always given the right to refuse to be floated to the AIDS unit. "When they try to float me to another unit," she says, "I respond that I can't go because I can't adequately meet the psychosocial needs of straight patients. But they usually float me anyway."

References

Ban on male nurses in labor and delivery is upheld. (1994). *RN,* *57*(12), 16.

Males win discrimination battle. (1992). *RN,* *55*(6), 16.

3

WORKING WITH COWORKERS AND MANAGERS

Be who you are. You don't need to jam it down people's throats. If you're friends, and comfortable with yourself, then talk about your partner. If it causes a problem, then you can fight or walk away. You decide if it's worth the fight to you.

An experienced lesbian nurse

The closet is no refuge, and it takes tremendous energy to maintain it. I have other uses for that energy.

A home health nurse

COMING OUT

The central question for many lesbian and gay nurses is whether to come out to their coworkers and boss. If they decide to come out, how will they do it? For some nurses, it is a moot point. "I've never once said I'm gay, or mentioned the word *boyfriend* or *significant other*. But everyone knows," says a gay man.

Although many nurses wish they could come out selectively to people they trust, gossip makes that impossible. "Because we work in a close environment, once you've come out to one person, you might as well come out to everybody," says a nurse on labor and delivery.

Why Come Out?

Some nurses come out for patient care reasons. They see a gay or lesbian patient receiving poor care because of prejudice or ignorance, and they come out while defending the patient. Others come out for personal, self-affirming reasons. "I made a decision that I needed to be out," says a psychiatric nurse. "I was getting sick in the closet." Most feel more genuine and energized after they come out. "Be out, you don't have to spend the energy to hide," says a lesbian who speaks for many people who have come out.

Nurses may come out because of a supportive environment. "It was open-minded, we knew everybody," says a newly out lesbian. "We served a diverse clientele, including gay people, so that made a difference."

Some nurses come out to stop the advances of single people at work. Says a young gay man, "One woman was attracted to me and I was certain that she was interested in me. She wanted to go to movies or to dinner together. I had to be careful not to lead her on. I'd drop hints that I was gay, and she eventually caught on." Another man teamed with a coworker. If a woman started to flirt, his female friend would take her aside and let her know that she was wasting her time.

Some nurses come out and urge others to come out as a way to improve conditions for all lesbian and gay nurses. They see themselves as role models for other gay and lesbian nurses and teachers for inexperienced heterosexual nurses. "Try to be quietly out, so that people see caring professionals who are gay," says a lesbian. Another woman agrees, "We all have an obligation to exercise some form of activism. Nurses are in a special position to open people's minds in a way that no one else can. But it's up to each nurse to measure the risk."

Another nurse explains, "To the extent that it feels safe, try to be out at work. The more visible we are, the more difficult it is for people to buy into the prejudice. If we put a face to the name (gay and lesbian), then people have to justify the hate laws."

Some nurses view coming out as an opportunity to correct stereotypes. "Gradually share your life with the people you work with, then they'll realize you're not much different than they are." Another nurse says coming out shows coworkers that, "we are just people who are doing a job."

Coming out enables some nurses to concentrate on larger professional issues. "Stop sweating the small stuff," says a gay man. "Some gay and lesbian nurses focus too much on the small stuff, and we need to see the bigger picture. If we keep our vision open and clear, then we can have an impact professionally."

Personal Empowerment

Many nurses focus on building quiet, yet sustaining, inner strength. "Believe in yourself, even though it can be difficult to do when you're different. Respect yourself." Another says, "Celebrate who you are without shame. There's nothing to hide from. The more people come out, the easier it will be."

This kind of strength allows nurses to fix on the issues they value. According to one woman, "We give people more power than they really have. If you concentrate on doing your own work, you'll be rewarded for it. You can't let things hold you back."

These nurses also recognize that the root of bigotry resides within the bigot, not the victim. "Work on your own self-acceptance. Let society work on its problem of not accepting gay and lesbian people. When we react to defend ourselves, we lose. Confront problems, then let go."

Another nurse agrees, "Be yourself, don't be ashamed of it. If they can't deal with it, that's their baggage. Don't waste time and energy worrying about what people think. It takes away from your clinical practice."

Deciding Not to Come Out

Coming out, however, can still result in physical and emotional dangers. Many experienced nurses do not assume that coworkers are friendly and trustworthy; instead, coworkers have to demonstrate these traits. "Get a feel for where you're at," says a staff nurse. "Are these the kind of people who are going to lynch you, or lie about you, because you're a lesbian?"

Sometimes the risk of coming out is too great. "I wasn't out period. It was a very scary town and institution," says a lesbian supervisor.

Some nurses decide not to come out at work under any circumstance. "I work the night shift, because no one talks about my social life. They're too busy working or talking about themselves," says a nurse working in an extended care facility. "Even if they did-n't fire you, they'd make it very difficult for you. I tell people that I was divorced many years ago, and they leave it alone."

Nurses who do not come out may spend considerable energy to ensure they remain hidden. "In jobs where I was really closeted, I couldn't even look another woman in the eye, for fear they would know."

Another lesbian who remained closeted for many years says, "Nurses get very close and talk about their boyfriends and husbands. For years I changed the pronouns when I talked about my relationships. I felt uncomfortable and prayed that they wouldn't ask specific questions."

At least one nurse does not come out because she fears it could impact patient care. "If I came out, I would be shunned socially, and that would be dangerous. If I needed help with a patient, they likely wouldn't help."

METHODS OF COMING OUT

The most common method nurses use to come out is to come out gradually by letting their coworkers know them as people first. A lesbian explains, "Initially I don't do anything. Through the general conversation I use my partner's name, and it allows people to sort it out for themselves. It's natural. It allows every-one as much time as they need to adjust."

A gay man elaborates, "I make people feel comfortable. I handle myself professionally and treat people ultrapolite. I don't talk about swing-from-the-chandelier sex in front of coworkers. The biggest thing that people can't get past is the sexual part. But I'm the stay-at-home, make-a-meat-loaf type."

Another nurse describes coming out in terms of intimacy, "Learn the social parameters, and don't live in fear of coming out. If you develop a level of intimacy with your coworkers or super-visor, then share your gay self."

A nurse who learned by experience adds, "When I came out, I decided to be out. I just announced it when I walked in the door. That wasn't so wise because it forced them to focus first on being gay. You've forced it to be a major issue, and it carries through the entire time they know you. Now I wait. When they have respect for my skills and knowledge, then being gay is a side issue."

An ICU nurse working in a small rural hospital came out by announcing that she was going to the Gay and Lesbian March on Washington in 1993. "They brought me out by asking about the march. I'm 42 years old, and I'm tired of pretending that I'm single and just not dating men."

Another nurse advises, "Get away from gender-neutral language. The world is changing. There's less need and reason to stay in the closet."

John, a young ICU nurse, came out gaily on National Coming Out Day, October 11. "I ordered three cakes decorated with rainbow flags saying 'Happy National Coming Out Day,' one for each shift. The card read, 'Thanks for liking me for the way I am.' I was tired of protecting my comments in front of other people, and assuming that my personal life didn't exist. No one had any negative comments." One nurse thanked him for his courage.

Supportive Coworkers

Several nurses are grateful for the support of their coworkers. Pam says, "It's a very small unit, so I shared with them as it was happening. One day I said, 'I kissed my first woman.'" Pam also used her colleagues to give her feedback, "When I questioned my choice later, they said, 'You seem much happier now than before.'"

Jean also found support from her coworkers, but the substance was different. "I work with a unique group of women. I feel real safe about being a lesbian at work. It doesn't feel like a challenge. People were waiting for me to come out. The manager was supportive and delighted. She saw it as the path for me. They all recognized that it was part of me finding my voice as a feminist."

A lesbian who was coming out remembers the importance of hearing encouraging words from her coworkers. One said, "That was a brave thing you did. I'm proud of you. I know I don't have to say this, but I want you to know that nothing will change at work." Another said, "I hope you'll still want to babysit my kids."

A nurse who is well liked by her peers thinks it is in part due to being in a committed relationship. "Because I have a partner and I'm wonderfully in love with her, so I'm not a threat to women."

Coworkers also show their support in other ways. In at least one hospital, nurses donated sick time to a gay nursing assistant with AIDS so that he could keep his health insurance.

A pediatric nurse describes the concern shown by her coworkers. "When my lover left me, everybody was supportive in an indirect way by asking me if I was OK or if I needed something. They let me know that they understood it was a tough time for me."

Coworkers Who Reject

Nurses in the early stages of coming out suffer when their coworkers make derogatory comments. A man who was not out to his coworkers recalls, "When someone gay is on the unit, you put up with so many jokes. And I had to deal with it indirectly by not coming out."

A nurse who was newly exploring her lesbian identity describes the difficulty disclosing to coworkers, "I felt isolated because I didn't feel that I could trust people from getting a look on their face—cloudy and stone-faced, that clinical look that you have an incurable disease. They don't want to get close because it might hurt them. It puts a wall up between us."

One woman describes how hard it was to socialize with heterosexual nurses because they rejected her. "It was OK when I went out with them, but they warned other women not to go with me because 'she's lesbian and will make a move on you.' They think that if you're gay, you're after every woman, and there's no discernment, like love doesn't count. I confronted them, but it didn't help. I left."

Many people assume that discrimination does not exist in San Francisco, but a nurse practitioner points out, "People on the east coast think of it as a Mecca. It's the most comfortable place to walk down the street holding hands, but even here there are hateful people who would say something if they weren't outnumbered by gays and lesbians. You pick who you come out to."

Closeted nurses hear a broader range of nonsensical, yet bigoted, comments from their coworkers. "The nurses on my shift were afraid that a gay orderly was passing AIDS to all the patients and attacking the women. They said that lesbians broke into the candy machine, and that gay people always hang out in the dark, so you can never find them."

After she realized she was lesbian, Kathy was more attuned to her coworkers' comments, and she turned to her union for help. "I was nervous, so I asked the union rep if I could be transferred. She was supportive, and told me to document any problems." Kathy decided not to come out to her coworkers because she did not feel it was a safe work environment. "People here don't even want to admit to being feminist. Women here feel it's more acceptable for a man to be gay than for a woman. The same generosity of spirit wouldn't be afforded me. I let them wonder." Yet she found an underlying sense of support, "The camaraderie of other women at work helped me through the difficult years of learning that I was a lesbian."

Table 3.1 *Homophobic Reactions to Lesbian Self-Disclosure* (Deevey, 1993) summarizes strategies for dealing with a wide variety of prejudiced remarks concerning coming out.

Feeling Like an Outsider

The culture on most nursing units is exclusively heterosexual, even when some of the nurses are not. The only sanctioned interests are mixed-gender dating, marriage, and children. This stifling culture keeps some in the closet. A staff nurse says:

> There's lots of gossip about whether this person is gay or that person is gay. Straight nurses talk about their relationships, but gay nurses don't bring it to work. It makes me feel very much like an outsider. You become close to the people you work with. These decisions don't build a good working rela-tionship. It's sad that my partner can't come and have lunch with me, when husbands stop in all the time. You have to be hush-hush, because they could use it against you.

Even after they come out, many gay and lesbian nurses feel separated from the people on their unit. A successful nurse explains:

> Being gay causes you problems daily, but not in the profound ways that people think of. But the discrimination is equally painful. People talk about social issues at lunch, but they don't talk about my issues, unless I make sure to bring it up. If I were a minority in a different category, I would be asked about my customs and holidays, but as a lesbian no one is interested in my customs. I have a sense of being different than others, but I can only integrate so far. I can function in both cultures, but I can only immerse myself in one culture.

Reaction	Private Response	Public Response
"You're a sinner."	The God Hates You Attack	"I respect your religious beliefs, but I insist that you treat me with respect."
"You're fired."	The Financial Ruin Attack	"This is a very emotional topic. Let's discuss it when we've both had a chance to think about this."
"Your mother/father was cold/sick/weak and caused you to be a lesbian."	The Child-of-Bad-Parents Attack	"We don't really know what causes either heterosexual or homosexual orientation. About 10% of all people are gay and lesbian, whatever their family background."
"You're an ugly woman who couldn't get a man."	The Body Image Attack	"Stereotypes about lesbians often include physical unattractiveness, man-hating, or lack of heterosexual experience, but none of these stereotypes is true."
"You should be ashamed—you bring danger/humiliation to this family/profession/neighborhood/nation."	The Guilt Trip Attack	"I am proud and happy to be a lesbian. I'd be glad to answer your questions about lesbian culture."
"I'll report you to the authorities. They'll take away your child."	The Unfit Mother Attack	"I am confident that I am a good parent to my child. She/he benefits from the courage and wisdom I have gained in dealing with my oppression as a lesbian."
"A patient complained to the head nurse that you asked him if he is gay. Why did you do that?"	The Professional Integrity Attack	"I believe each patient should be asked about sexual orientation to make clear that we offer good care to *all* patients."
"I'll tell your partner's parents/employer/grandmother."	The Attack on the Closeted Partner	"You can threaten me with scandal, but blackmail is illegal, and I will sue you."
"Are you the little boy or the little girl?"	The Lesbians-as-Pseudo-Heterosexuals Attack	(Some questions I don't dignify with an answer.)

TABLE 3.1   Homophobic Reactions to Lesbian Self-Disclosure

Reaction	Private Response	Public Response
"It's OK with me if you're a lesbian, so long as you keep your hands off my neck."	The Predatory Lesbian Attack	"We lesbians make pretty clear distinctions between courting and friendship with women. I think you'll continue to feel safe with me."
"You mean all this time you didn't tell me? Why don't you trust me?"	The Lesbians-Are-Liars Attack	"Try to imagine for the next 48 hours that you are a lesbian. It takes courage and compromise to survive in a hostile environment."
"You're so comfortable talking about lesbian issues. I can't believe you get angry or scared about homophobia."	The Looks-So-Easy Attack	"I do accept myself. But the world is still hostile and violent toward gay and lesbian people. I never can predict if I'll be safe in a new situation."
"There's no reason to do research on lesbian women, no need to provide special services. You have convinced me that lesbian women are no different from other women."	The Denial of Difference Attack	"It's true that lesbian women are not 'different' in the sense of being emotionally disturbed or sinful or criminal. But the prejudice against us causes minority stress and has generated a hidden lesbian culture that few straight people know about."
"When you get AIDS, I'll take care of you."	The So-Much-to-Learn Attack	"Lesbian women are actually the lowest-risk population for AIDS; but I appreciate your support."
"You're disgusting and sick."	The Blatant Attack	"I see you have a problem. I'd be glad to recommend a good therapist."
"I never met one before."	The Honest Truth Response— one I respect.	"Well, you're in luck. If you want to know more about gay and lesbian culture, I love to answer questions. I've been asked all kinds of things, so don't be shy."

TABLE 3.1 Homophobic Reactions to Lesbian Self-Disclosure (continued)

From "Lesbian self-disclosure strategies for success," by S. Deevey. *Journal of Psychosocial Nursing,* 1993, Vol. 31, No. 4. Reprinted with permission.

Sally's Coworkers Rejected Her

Although they had worked together for years and ostensibly respected her as a nurse and as a married woman, Sally's coworkers rejected her when she came out. "It was a shock. They had a rugged time. I trusted them too much, and I must have threatened them, because I used to be like them. One friend told me, 'I'm so disappointed in you. I admired you. You taught me everything, you have a perfect family.' I felt shamed."

It was hard for her to deal with her coworkers' stereotypical questions. "They asked if I was attracted to all women. I said, 'Yes, I love women, but working here isn't an emotional experience.'"

Friendships dissolved. Sally remembers, "Some of my friends didn't want to talk to me. Another wanted to cure me. Another woman tried to hit on me. She had a family, and I felt guilty."

Her work performance was scrutinized without justification. "For years I had been looked up to. I precepted the new nurses. Suddenly, I was under a microscope. I got called into the office every other day. Suddenly, my charting wasn't right. Or if I told a joke, now they just stared at me, no one laughed. The easy camaraderie you need to work together was lost."

BEING OUTED

Because of discrimination and stigma, almost all lesbians and gay men want to control who knows. Because there are potential physical and emotional risks from coming out, only the individual can judge whether the benefits outweigh the risks.

When someone else discloses your sexual orientation, it is called outing. Outing can be very unsettling even when the intention is friendly. An ICU nurse who was newly dealing with her identity remembers when two coworkers guessed that she was a lesbian, "They asked, and I acknowledged. I was very scared at first. I thought they'd out me to the whole unit, and administration would find some reason to get rid of me."

The risk of being outed may feel so great that it causes nurses to change jobs. "In another place where I worked, a nurse that I worked with let it be known that I was gay because she was gay too," says a staff nurse. "It was very uncomfortable for me. It's one of the reasons why I left."

Because so many nurses gossip about their coworkers, they do not even realize when they out someone. A staff nurse recalls, "First I came out to the people I knew, then it spread like wildfire. Some people talked behind my back."

Dealing with Outing

Being outed can happen suddenly and feel shocking. People upset by being outed may need support right away by talking with a supervisor or a lesbian or gay coworker or friend. Jim Lovette, a gay nurse and a psychotherapist, suggests that people use the distress of being outed as an opportunity to explore their beliefs and support networks. "We all have moments of negative feelings about ourselves as gay people," says Lovette. "Our internal bigot is worse than the social bigot that calls you names."

First, examine why you are closeted.

What was upsetting about being outed?

What do you believe about yourself in terms of being lesbian or gay?

Is it unsafe to be out at work?

What are the legal ramifications of being outed? Being outed in the military, for example, has different consequences, than being outed in a hospital that prohibits discrimination.

If it is unsafe to be out at work, why do you keep the job? Do the benefits outweigh the distress of remaining closeted?

Is remaining closeted a self-imposed standard?

How do coworkers, especially other lesbian and gay coworkers, deal with personal information?

What was the social context in which the outing occurred? Was it a request by a potential friend to become closer, or was it really a weapon intended to cause pain?

Will you have an ongoing relationship, such as with a coworker, or a time-limited relationship, such as with a patient?

"Sexual orientation in this culture is not an entirely private matter," says Lovette. "It may be appropriate to acknowledge your sexual orientation at work. If you passively or actively deny that you're gay, you reinforce the invisibility of being gay and feed into the myth that all people are straight."

If the outing was intended as harassment, you may have recourse through your supervisor. "If you don't challenge bigotry, then you're empowering it," says Lovette. Outing and coming out are recurrent issues.

If, for reasons of personal, emotional, or physical safety, you need to defend yourself from being exposed, focus on the process instead of the answer. You might ask, "Why is this important now? Why do you want to know?" It forces the person to defend his or her question, rather than you defending your answer.

"When you're out, you're in charge of the information that goes out about you. It's very empowering," says Lovette.

Supportive Managers

Several nurses describe managers who bent the rules to help lesbian and gay nurses. "My partner had cancer," remembers a lesbian. "My boss let me have time off to be with her when she was in a crisis. The supervisor let me take sick time or vacation time off." Another woman says, "When my previous lover died, my nurse manager gave me bereavement leave for her funeral."

Janet, a nurse manager, got support for her relationship which was stressed by her long hours at work. She explains, "I also got tired of being expected to work extra because I was single and didn't have a family to go home to. My partner can get just as mad and scream just as loud as any husband when I bring work home."

Because Janet was out to her director, they could talk about the real issues. "One time I came to my director in tears because

I couldn't get home on time, and my partner was complaining about my 12-hour days, and she wanted time for our relationship. The director was supportive and talked to me for an hour about my feelings and things that I could try in order to get home earlier. She told me, 'We need you here, but she needs you too.'"

USING STAGES OF COMING OUT

Wise supervisors know how to structure the work environment to encourage the best performance and morale from employees. This task is more complicated for gay men and lesbians because each person's needs are in part determined by his or her stage of coming out, which changes over time. The Cass (1979) six-stage model of coming out may help.

Stage 1: Identity Confusion

Nurses in this stage need positive role models and an environment free of prejudice. It is important to describe people as individuals rather than as cultural stereotypes. They also need an environment free of gossip and pejorative jokes.

Stage 2: Identity Comparison

Besides role models and an environment free of prejudice, people in this stage need kindness and understanding. They may be moody, and even an innocent question such as, "Do you have a boyfriend?" may be vexing because they do not want to reveal themselves. They simultaneously need friendship and distance. They probably avoid discussing relationships, love, or sex. They still feel very threatened by gossiping and pejorative joking, because they feel that they are being secretly judged.

Stage 3: Identity Tolerance

People in this stage seek reassurance that they are still admired for their personal traits and respected for their professional skills. They want to know that they are still the same, yet different and growing. Work may provide an anchor to stability. This is the time for sincere compliments, especially about work-related skills. They may want a clear delineation between work and social relationships.

Stage 4: Identity Acceptance

At this stage, people love to talk about their life, loves, and insights. They need nonjudgmental, yet curious, listeners. Work may not be as important as it once was because of the conflicting time demands of a personal life.

Stage 5: Identity Pride

At this stage, political activism may become important. For example, gay and lesbian nurses might be outraged because there are no benefits for same-sex domestic partners. It may be a good time for certain committee work. They must have Gay Pride Day off. They insist on wearing symbols of lesbian or gay identity, and they feel a terrible injustice in being counseled not to wear them. They may need to be reminded that coworkers are entitled to their own political opinions, and work may not be the best place for a political discussion. They need to know that the rules are consistently and fairly applied.

Stage 6: Identity Synthesis

People in this final stage demonstrate a unique maturity. Because they know exactly who they are, they can respect and be present for others. At the same time, they know how to avoid or upbraid bigots and fools. They need a job that is challenging and respects their lifestyle and talents. Although they may be activists, they are far better able to pick their battles and form coalitions.

DISCRIMINATION

For too many lesbian and gay nurses, discrimination is real. When coworkers discriminate, gay and lesbian nurses get too little support from their supervisors because their complaints are dismissed as personality conflicts. When managers discriminate, it denies qualified nurses the promotions they deserve. Lesbian and gay nurses frequently respond by transferring to another unit or quitting. How much experience has been lost because of discrimination? How much money is needlessly spent to train their replacements?

Discrimination by Coworkers

Coworkers may display their rejection of gay and lesbian nurses through discrimination. A lesbian says, "When I came out, they were shocked initially. Some were angry, and I got bad assignments. They wouldn't direct comments directly at me."

A nurse who works midnights reports, "One of the nurses said she didn't want to come in on nights because she didn't want to be alone with me. The boss was a fundamentalist and didn't reprimand the nurse."

Discrimination by Managers

The prejudice is often left unsaid, or nurses are reprimanded for vague complaints. A student intern explains, "The staff educator said that some of the nurses aides complained that I was different and not fitting in, that I needed to be more friendly. It was weird. I thought that it might be because I'm gay, but no one confronted me." By focusing on the intern's personality, the educator proved that she was more interested in harassing the intern than improving her performance.

Even experienced nurses are left to question their skills or self-esteem because prejudice is unstated. A nurse explains, "The charge nurse thing didn't happen when it should, and it wasn't because of my skills. I never was given a chance. For years, I thought I wasn't living up to their standards; but in retrospect, I think I did meet the standards, and it was discrimination. Because I wasn't on the road to getting married and having babies like 95% of the nurses at that hospital."

Sometimes discrimination affects patient assignments. One nurse describes her situation:

> Every night I got the worst assignment. The charge nurse would get the three MI patients who slept through the night, while I got the patients who had TPN, needed blood, and had diarrhea. When I signed out for overtime, the charge

nurse would give me attitude and asked me why I worked so slow. When I left, I felt totally empty, without a shred of self-esteem. I felt like I was run over by a truck that then backed over me, and ran over me again. I didn't work as a nurse as long as I could.

Bart describes a series of incidents:

I had a charge nurse, a preacher's wife who was evil and hateful. She looked like she wouldn't spit on me if I was burning. I always suspected that it was because I was gay, but I'll never know. She'd follow behind me to double-check my work, and hover over me. I was never assigned the teenage boys or young men. I always got the little old ladies. I didn't confront her directly about the assignments because it would be used against me to show that I was trying to get at a patient. The woman had worked there since God was a small child. I brought it up to the director of nursing, who said many people had personality conflicts with my charge nurse. She didn't openly deal with the gay issues, even though she knew I was gay. Instead she transferred me off the unit.

Margaret suspects that she was discriminated against. "I was out to the supervisor, and I was denied advancement in the clinical ladder. She used the fact that I worked nights to deny the advancement. But another person on nights was advanced. Shortly after that, I left the unit."

A minor but obvious form of discrimination involves holiday requests. In many places, the first choice goes to people with families, but lesbian and gay families are not recognized. Instead, gay and lesbian nurses are considered single and without needs during the holidays.

A gay man describes how his manager prejudiced his coworkers even before he arrived: "I worked in a dialysis unit, where people treated me odd. Finally, the social worker told me that the head nurse had a meeting with the staff before I came to tell them that I was gay, and I couldn't work with certain patients, because it would cause problems. She had the management style of a barbarian. She was never satisfied with what I did and screamed at me on the unit."

Instead of quitting, he tried to find a solution within the system. "First I went to the director of nursing and the director of human resources. After that, the head nurse changed, and I could do no wrong. But I was never comfortable. There was no way to undo what had been done."

Another gay man complains, "Everyone stuck their nose in my business whenever I called in sick, they wanted desperately to know my HIV status, but they wouldn't ask outright."

Gay and lesbian nurses are also influenced by how other lesbian and gay people are treated. A staff nurse resigned because a gay assistant director was mistreated. She explains, "They cleaned out his desk. There were people with trash cans throwing away his personal stuff. If they treated him that way, how would they treat me?"

Discrimination by Doctors

Several gay men describe doctors who behave very unprofessionally by bashing. One man recalls, "Physicians are more threatened by male nurses, and they use the sexual orientation issue to undermine you as a professional colleague. I've been called names. I say, 'So what? Now let's get back to the real issue.'"

Although some coworkers are supportive, too often they tacitly support bashing. "Everybody disappears because they don't want to deal with it," says a man who has been bashed publicly. "The people who shrink into the wallpaper undercut me as a gay nurse and nursing as a whole."

PREJUDICE BASED ON SECTARIAN BELIEFS

One of the most common complaints of gay and lesbian nurses involves discrimination by coworkers who hold sectarian religious convictions. Their quarrel is not with religion, but with the narrow-minded harassment committed in its name. Jim's complaints are typical. "I worked with a woman who told me that being gay was a sin and that I was going to hell because of it. I complained to the director who should have fired her but didn't. The director sided with her because they both belonged to the same church. I eventually quit." Over and over, lesbian and gay nurses report that their only recourse is to transfer or quit.

Henry describes a nurse who took her prejudice another step. After delivering the going-to-hell sermon, she continued to undermine his position at the hospital. "She tried to get me fired by making up stories that I was making sexual advances toward patients, which of course wasn't true. She also told some of the patients that I was gay."

Brenda Is Insulted

Well-meaning, but prejudiced, sectarians may not recognize the suffering they cause. They do not understand that although their concerns for a gay or lesbian's soul may be sincere, their seemingly kind words still hit like fists. Brenda tells of a well-meaning coworker who confronted her during a break in the nurse's lounge. This story will sound familiar to most out lesbian and gay nurses.

Coworker: "Tell me, do you believe in God?"

Brenda (from behind her newspaper): "Yeah."

Coworker: "Then how do you justify the way you live?"

Brenda: "Please don't insult me. I don't want to have this conversation here."

Coworker: "I'm not trying to insult you."

Brenda: "But you are, and I don't want to talk about it here."

Later Brenda recalls, "I stumbled through it in the lounge without losing my composure, but when I got home I had a good cry. I expect the place I work to be safe, and I suddenly felt very vulnerable." Although Brenda intended to forget the incident, her manager heard about it through the grapevine and offered her support. The coworker was formally disciplined for interfering with Brenda's ability to work and interfering with the provision of a safe work environment. The issues were correctly reframed from religious freedom to harassment.

It turned out to be a growth experience for both nurses. The coworker later offered a heart-felt apology. Brenda says, "On another occasion, I told her that I enjoyed working with her, and she was moved. There was a general sense of forgiveness, and we acknowledged a new level of respect for one another."

This situation illustrates that anyone can be a target. Although Brenda is a highly respected nurse, she was still harassed. It is based on the prejudices of the offender, rather than the merits of the victim. Second, the system of progressive discipline can work. You have more options than transferring or quitting. In addition, confrontation can lead to a greater understanding, not just hard feelings.

Advice from an MCC Minister

Universal Fellowship of Metropolitan Community Churches (MCC) was started in 1968 to offer gay and lesbian Christians a place to worship and participate in the full life of the congregation. MCC is still denied membership in the Metropolitan Council of Churches, but boasts over 32,000 members worldwide. According to Reverend Judy Gingerich, a former nurse and a pastor of the MCC church in Charlottesville, "These people believe so strongly, that makes it a challenge. But it's harassment, even if they think it's helping." For Gingerich, "Part of God's truth is knowing who we are as gay and lesbian people, then it becomes a life-giving source for us." She offers the following advice to nurses who are confronted at work:

- ▾ If you are confronted publicly, say, "Can we talk about it later privately; for example, at lunch. It's inappropriate to talk about this in front of the patient." This allows you time to prepare and calm down.

- ▾ Remind a Christian, "There are no words from Jesus about homosexuality."

- ▾ If the person quotes Bible verses, say, "I understand that we see scripture from a different point of view, so it won't benefit us to argue about scripture. If you want to discuss something else, that's OK."

- ▾ If the person insists on quoting scripture, then refer to any passage spelling out God's love for all of us, such as Galatians 3:28.

- ▾ If the person offers to pray for you, respond by saying, "Thank you, I can always use prayer. I'll pray for you too."

▾ Try to keep the discussion focused on the right of everyone to have personal religious beliefs. Say, "Is it possible for us to agree to disagree? That doesn't mean that I don't respect you."

Gingerich offers a final note of caution, "Don't get caught up in the trap of getting all your energy sucked out by an argument. We use so much energy defending ourselves from people who are trying to ruin us, when we could be using that energy to help people."

Advice from a Lesbian Christian

Debra is now a deacon in MCC, as well as a nurse. But she came to her religious beliefs the hard way. "Having been raised in a hard-sell fundamentalist Baptist church, and struggling with my sexuality, and feeling that having sex with a woman was the worst sin you can do, and botching several suicide attempts, I now have a deeper understanding."

God still plays a central role in her life. "I have a deal with God. I don't lie to God, and he or she doesn't lie to me. And being straight would be a lie for me. When I stand before my maker, I will be able to say that I lived my life with as full an understanding of who I am as I am capable."

When confronted with possible harassment, Debra first determines whether a person is a "real Christian" or just judgmental. "Christians are people who want to better the world because they care about people. They believe that you're missing out, and they want you to have a personal walk with God, and you can't do that, in their eyes, if you're gay. But real Christians look at other people's lives and want them to be full. I've never had a problem with a real Christian." Debra will discuss her beliefs and quote scripture with "real Christians."

On the other hand, she steers clear of the egotistically judgmental. "There are other people who want you to believe exactly like them, and if you don't, then you're bad. They think that they're better than you. They're never going to understand, and I don't waste my time with them." One of her favorite passages from the Bible starts with Matthew 7:1, "Judge not, that ye be not judged."

Like many gay and lesbian nurses, she finds support and solace from her Christian beliefs. "I want to be treated as a human being who counts, and that's how God wants me to treat others, and to be treated."

MILITARY NURSES

The military has a long, but largely untold, history of gay and lesbian nurses. According to one Vietnam-era veteran, "About 75% of the Nurse Corp was lesbian or gay during the war. Once they let pregnant nurses stay, it all changed. Now it's the opposite."

The military confronts gay and lesbian nurses with contradictions. Initially, it offers a great sense of freedom, an acceptable way for young men and women to leave home, take adult responsibilities, gain advanced training, and see the world. Many are drawn by a system that puts women in the company of many other women, and men in the company of other men. One woman says, "The military is really into sports as a way to build morale; and those women's softball teams, oh my God. Most of our team was straight, but the other teams were mostly gay. What a great way to spend time with women."

Because they are single and more flexible, gay men and lesbians easily move up the ranks. They praise the military for the opportunities it offers, especially for advanced practice. One military nurse says, "I truly enjoy serving my country. In the military, I can be a leader. I have more autonomy. Nurses are the glue that holds everything together, and we're allowed to think. Because of the ranking system, the head nurse may have a higher rank than the physician. I tried civilian nursing, and you can't get this role as a civilian."

But they also complain of the need to hide their sexual orientation. Explains one officer, "At home I have my gay life, and when I put on my military uniform, I'm straight." Another nurse agrees, "At work you don't talk about your social life. You become a Dr. Jekyll and Mr. Hyde."

Blackmail in the Military

Blackmail is far more of a threat in the military than in civilian life. "I never tell my straight friends in the military that I'm gay, because they can use it against me," says an experienced nurse. "You really have to watch your back, because as you get up there higher in rank, someone who is under scrutiny will cash in their friends to try to save themselves."

A gay nurse illustrates this point with an example involving sexual indiscretion. "A friend of mine was attracted to a young, enlisted LPN who was very immature. The LPN started to get in trouble for other problems, like not coming to work. When he saw that he was sinking, he decided to take someone with him; and my friend lost his career."

One man described an alcoholic corpsman who tried to blackmail him in exchange for a soft work life. The nurse firmly responded, "You will do what I assign you to do. This is how you will deal with me: my personal life doesn't affect you." The charge nurse was supportive, and the threats of blackmail stopped.

Because the miliary attracts and promotes competitive people, the threat of blackmail increases with each promotion. "In today's military, with downsizing, there are fewer opportunities, so there's more cutthroat behavior," explains a gay man. An officer describes how a friend was victimized. "She was blackmailed by a heterosexual who wanted her job. She was moved out of a supervisory position, and three months later, she was shipped overseas. In short, they got rid of her."

A veteran nurse explains how the system works:

In Vietnam, I worked in a MASH unit, like the TV show. A nurse who reported to me came on duty drunk as a skunk. There was no way she could do her job safely, so I made her go off duty. She went to the authorities and accused me of being a lesbian. That started a complete investigation. They played "good cop, bad cop" just like on TV when they interrogated me. They kept asking me if I knew anyone who was a lesbian. The way it works is they make a report, but only the commanding officer can press charges. In this case, the commanding officer was the Chief Nurse, who was also a lesbian. She called me into her office and looked up from the report. First she asked me if I had slept with the nurse who was sent off duty, as if the real problem might be jealousy. I told her that I hadn't. She put down the report and said, "There, but for the grace of God, go I." And she told me that she wasn't going to press charges. I also know that she respected my partner at the time, and she watched out for us.

"Don't Ask, Don't Tell"

In 1993, Congress approved President Clinton's so-called "don't ask, don't tell" policy, which allows gay men and lesbians to serve in the armed forces as long as they hide their sexual orientation and do not engage in homosexual conduct, which includes obvious sexual acts, as well as innocent displays of affection. The policy also assumes that if you admit you are lesbian or gay, you will also engage in sexual misconduct and must be discharged. Touted by Clinton as a reform, it replaced a total ban on gays and lesbians in the military. Explains a gay nurse who has served under both policies, "Under 'don't ask, don't tell,' you can go to gay bars, but you can't dance together, and you can't hold hands. Everyone is breathing easier. If I do my job, no one cares what I do at home. The days of witch hunts are dying, but not gone."

Not everyone reports the same degree of freedom. "Because I'm highly visible in my role, I can't go to gay or lesbian bars, because I don't want to jeopardize my position and all I've worked for by being seen. The military police will do a witch hunt by cruising the parking lot of a gay bar looking for military tags."

The distinctions between earlier forms of discrimination and the current "don't ask, don't tell" policy do not go far enough to satisfy everyone. Says one Army nurse, "It's a big joke, a big lie. It's like putting a Band-Aid on a gaping wound. It was really a way to chapter out gays and lesbians."

In March 1995, a federal judge ruled that "don't ask, don't tell" violates the free-speech and equal-protection rights of gay men and lesbians. U.S. District Court Judge Eugene Nickerson delivered a harshly worded 39-page decision denouncing the policy as pandering to the prejudices of heterosexuals.

Personal Cost in the Military

The most obvious cost gay and lesbian nurses pay for remaining in the military is the loss of relationships with lovers. Explains one lesbian, "When we separated after a six-year relationship, I didn't have anyone to talk to about how I felt. I blame the military for putting so much distance between us. There just wasn't anything left to our relationship."

A gay man echoes the difficulty of finding and keeping a lover, "I've had a lot of fun being on active duty, but having a long-term lover has suffered. The military is a demanding career, and that's also had an effect. But I don't know if I use the military as an excuse."

Fake Husbands, Fake Wives

Many gay and lesbian nurses effectively hide in the military by pretending to be heterosexuals. "About half of the gay and lesbian nurses have arranged marriages, especially the paranoid ones," says an Army nurse. "Because of unaccompanied tours of duty, you don't even have to live together. You get extra pay, medical benefits, PX benefits, and officers can even move off base."

Explains one gay nurse, "When I came on active duty, my female roommate wanted to go to Europe. So we got married, and it was a good cover. We stayed married for several years, until she found a man she really wanted to marry. It worked for both of us."

DEALING WITH CONFLICT

Outside the military, nurses and their managers have more options for dealing with conflicts caused by bigoted remarks.

How Bette Handles Conflicts

Bette was recruited into her nurse manager position and has been out to her boss and coworkers for years. She describes how to intervene in staff conflicts:

> I only step in if someone makes a derogatory comment, but otherwise I don't make an issue. I think we tolerate far too much in nursing in terms of personality conflicts. You have to deal with conflicts openly. I intervene if I notice that they're not helping each other, or if another staff member tells me about a conflict. I talk to them separately about what the real issues are and are not. If their real issues are gay and lesbian issues, then they have

to deal with it. I tell them, "I don't care if you like each other, but you have to work together, or one of you needs to make a change or find a new job." If they can't reconcile working with gay nurses, then I'd counsel the person with the problems to make a change or look at another position or another unit. I can't see penalizing the gay employee for someone else's narrow-mindedness. If the person is hiding behind being gay and the real problem is performance, then I'd set goals.

Although supportive of lesbian and gay employees, she does not define herself exclusively in terms of being lesbian. "I see myself as being gay, yes, but it's not all encompassing. When I'm at work, I don't need to talk about if Jesse Helms is right or wrong."

Confronting Bigotry

Gay and lesbian nurses must decide whether to confront their coworker's prejudiced comments. Frequent confrontations can be draining and alienating; yet allowing bigotry to go unchallenged tacitly supports discrimination. An experienced nurse explains, "I've heard snide comments behind my back, and I usually let it pass. I try not to get involved with defending myself. I decide in my mind what is right and just, then I get involved."

A lesbian nurse describes a confrontation she had with a coworker:

> I ripped up a woman on our unit who complained about the (*very offensive slang for gay men*) who spread AIDS. I had just lost a friend at church (who died of AIDS) and I let her know that she was wrong and mean to boot. She backed down and no one else interfered. The next day I came back to her and apologized for losing my temper. But I only apologized for the way I said it, not what I said.

Closeted nurses face the additional dilemma of whether confronting injustice will force them to come out. Many have learned to address injustice on humanitarian grounds. An out lesbian nurse offers advice:

Weigh carefully when you confront someone, because you're vulnerable, and the stakes are high. Walk away until you increase your power base. You don't want to pay more than you can afford to pay. When I feel degraded about the distorted remarks, I can confront the distortion, and not come out as a gay person. Some people feel trapped by not being able to come out entirely. The question belongs to the person who asks it, the answer belongs to you. And you can choose to make the answer as connected to the question as you want to.

WORKING WITH LESBIAN AND GAY NURSES

Other gay and lesbian nurses at work can be a pleasure or a frustration. For some, the closet prevents them from associating with other gay or lesbian nurses. Still others choose their friends for reasons that are independent of sexual orientation. But a large number of nurses seek out the company of other lesbian and gay people at work.

For many, friendship seems easier, deeper, and longer lasting with other gay or lesbian people. "I love working with gay people. It's much more fun to have a soulmate. You can say little things just for fun, and they automatically understand. They can cut to the chase. Straight people don't ever really get it."

Some nurses describe a stronger team effort with other lesbian or gay nurses. "Other gay nurses pull for you," says an ICU nurse. "Dorothy (another lesbian nurse) and I had an understanding that she would deal with the phlegm, and I'd deal with the stool and vomit."

A gay man agrees, "You cut them more slack, and you're more willing to be there for each other. You can work like a hand-in-glove rapport because there's a kinship there."

A lesbian who works in a small rural hospital says, "There's a gay orderly who also works midnights; and knowing that he's in the building makes me feel like there's family here. Sometimes we cross in the hall and hug each other."

One woman feels that other lesbian nurses also help her with patient care. "A lesbian surgical nurse gave me a very good patient report. When I get pulled to a unit with lesbian nurses, they give me extra time and attention."

The Closet Community

Newly out nurses must learn through trial and error how to deal with the closet community. A nurse describes her first two years of lesbian experience:

> I thought in coming out that I would be welcomed and have an automatic connection—but it's not true. It's frustrating. People complain that there are so many gay people at work, when there's really only a few. Several nurses are lesbians, who are relatively out, and thrilled that I was coming out. But, many lesbian nurses are leading very traditional lives, have a house, aren't out, and are very happy. I need to recognize that there's a lot of diversity among gay and lesbian people and that's good.

An ICU nurse remembers, "Being out has distanced me from people who aren't out. Most avoid me like the plague. They're scared, because they think no one knows."

Closeted managers may even discriminate against openly lesbian or gay nurses. A lesbian who was denied a promotion says, "I had a manager who I suspected of discrimination because she was uncomfortable with my openness around my sexual orientation. I almost felt that it made her uncomfortable because it was the life she wished she had been brave enough to lead."

The closet may extend outside of work. "I saw another nurse who I suspected was a lesbian at the Gay Pride Parade," says a staff nurse. "For months she avoided me because she thought I would talk about gay rights."

A LESBIAN OR GAY BOSS

Some nurses seek another gay man or lesbian as a boss. A woman working in an outpatient clinic says, "Because my supervisor is gay, I have an ongoing, gratifying relationship. It's great to come to work with another out nurse."

Some people might assume that gay and lesbian employees expect preferential treatment from a lesbian or gay boss. It usually does not happen. A supervisor says, "The other five or ten gay employees don't expect anything differently from me because I'm gay."

But a nurse manager in the South had a different experience with a gay employee who took liberties. The manager explains, "He thought that because we share this thing that others don't, I should be more lenient." The manager strives not to play favorites and undermine the unit's morale. He also wants to apply appropriate disciplinary actions. "I grapple with overreacting or being too harsh," he admits. "It's hard to set appropriate boundaries because we know one another on a different level."

Even when the boss and a substantial number of coworkers are lesbian and gay, the supervisor may not feel comfortable being completely out. Says a former nurse manager of an AIDS unit, "Because I was the boss, there's a separation between the boss and the worker. The defined expectations of decorum prevented me from being fully out."

DATING AT WORK

For heterosexuals, work is a common place to meet prospective marriage partners, and few large companies regulate dating among employees. How do gay and lesbian nurses date at work?

An out gay pediatric nurse remembers how his coworkers respected his socializing at work. "We usually ate as a group. But one day they sat away from me when they saw that I was having an intimate conversation with another man. Later, they admitted that they wanted to see me find someone special. It felt very warm and natural."

A lesbian complained that her coworkers were trying to prevent her from dating. "I was going out to a movie with a student and the staff felt compelled to warn her that I was gay," she explains. "First I talked about it with my boss and she agreed that I confront them. I said, 'This needs to stop right here and now. What I do on my own time is my own business.'"

A gay nurse manager of an AIDS unit that attracts many gay and lesbian nurses complains about inappropriate socializing. "Some gay nurses are indiscreet with doctors and too familiar with patients, and use work as a way to get dates. It meets the negative stereotype, and I think we're much more than that."

WORKING WITH YOUR PARTNER

Many large companies regulate how married partners work together. They usually cannot work in the same department, and one partner never supervises another. But gay and lesbian people are usually immune from these rules, because they are written with a heterosexual bias. Should the same rules apply to same-gender relationships?

Margaret thinks the same rules should apply. She worked on a close-knit specialty unit with her lover. "It made it more awkward and was part of the reason I left. You reach a certain point where it's time for one of you to leave."

A manager describes the difficulties he had supervising his lover. "It meant that our personal fights spilled over into work. When things were good, they were very good; but when things were bad, they were terrible."

Lisa and her partner work on the same floor without difficulty. "Married people can work together here, it doesn't cause us a problem to work together." How do they make it work? "We agree not to talk about work at home, and the difference in our shifts allows us time home alone."

Most experienced managers would strongly recommend that lovers refrain from working on the same shift of the same unit, and that lovers avoid supervisor-employee relationships. Eventually it will cause problems, and the victim could be your relationship.

COPING

Nursing is a stressful profession, and being gay or lesbian compounds the stress. How do nurses deal with the stress?

- ▾ "I've mastered the art of leaving work at work. I work hard at work, and play hard at home."

- ▾ "I go to a support group at the gay community center twice a week. We're almost a family."

- ▾ "Having a life outside of nursing and having friends who have nothing to do with medicine."

▼ "Subscribe to gay and lesbian publications."

▼ "My own belief system is helpful, my religious convictions."

▼ "Exercise. I also coach a basketball team."

▼ "Have a good girlfriend (or boyfriend)."

▼ "Keep your sense of humor."

▼ "Spending time with my lover and my animals."

▼ "Spend time alone."

▼ "Have a small group of friends who you're out to. They are vital, they can take your side. It's like having an army behind you."

SUMMARY

Although many nurses support and admire their lesbian and gay coworkers, discrimination remains a real threat. It either robs nurses of the pleasure of working, or prevents them from being promoted. A few gay and lesbian nurses seek justice through their employer's grievance process, but most victims of discrimination leave. Training their replacements is expensive. Because of discrimination, lesbian and gay nurses may be afraid to come out. In a profession that claims to value the diversity of patients, it is sadly ironic that there is so little respect for the diversity of its practitioners.

References

Cass, V. C. (1979). Homosexual identity formation: A theoretical model. *Journal of Homosexuality, 4*(5), 219–235.

Deevey, S. (1993). Lesbian self-disclosure strategies for success. *Journal of Psychosocial Nursing, 31*(4), 21–26.

4 | LEGAL ISSUES

*Now our department has a policy of nondiscrimina-
tion on the basis of sexual orientation, and that's a
direct result of my grievance.*

Bill, a nurse unfairly denied promotion

CONSTANT AND UNPREDICTABLE CHANGES

We think of civil rights as fundamental and equally applied across
the country, but lesbians and gay men have fewer rights than do
other Americans. Legal protections exist only in small pockets
across the country and the extent of protections varies widely.
Civil rights for lesbians and gay men are changing rapidly, but
not always in the direction of respecting the rights of all
Americans. The U.S. Supreme Court, which in the past has
refused to hear many cases concerning gay men and lesbians,
faces several key appeals.

Because the federal government has failed to take a leadership position for gay and lesbian rights, by default, the most influential decisions are made by voters in state and local elections.
Sometimes the voters endorse equal rights, sometimes they take
rights away. Many voter decisions—both in favor of equal rights
and restricting human rights—are challenged in court. Decisions
in court in one state may contradict decisions made in another
state, and rulings frequently change on appeal.

Many observers predict that equal rights for gay men and lesbians will replace abortion issues as the most deftly tossed political football of the next decade. Unfortunately, the discussion of lesbian and gay rights contains few facts and too many half-truths and self-serving rhetoric. Reporting on gay and lesbian issues is usually incomplete and inaccurate. Instead, the media too often repeats societal bigotry against gay men and lesbians.

People who deny basic civil rights to lesbians and gay men frequently use the propaganda slogan "special rights" to justify their bigotry. They argue that protecting gay men and lesbians from discrimination in housing, employment, education, and public accommodation will grant them more rights than are extended to all other Americans. In truth, lesbians and gay men are struggling to reach parity. Special rights also illustrates "heterosexism," the belief that heterosexuality is the only proper orientation, and people who behave otherwise deserve to be punished. They view lesbian, gay, or bisexual orientations as a preference that could be changed, rather than a biological imperative. They argue that lesbians, gay men, and bisexuals can end discrimination by forcing themselves to be heterosexuals or by hiding.

NO FEDERAL PROTECTION

Many people are surprised that federal law does not already prohibit discrimination against gay men and lesbians solely on the basis of sexual orientation. On the federal level, it is legal to discriminate on the basis of sexual orientation and deny lesbians and gay men jobs, housing, public accommodation, access to education, and entrance into the military. Federal laws do not protect gay men and lesbians from being fired solely because of sexual orientation.

The Federal Government as an Employer

The federal government protects lesbians and gay men better as an employer than as government. Some people are protected from discrimination on the basis of sexual orientation by agency policies. According to the National Gay & Lesbian Task Force (1994), the following agencies bar discrimination: the Federal Bureau of Investigation, the Department of the Interior, the Justice Department, the White House, the Department of Housing and Urban Development, the Department of Transportation, the Office of Personnel Management, and the State Department. As employees in these agencies, lesbians and gay men can formally grieve discriminatory practices based on sexual orientation.

THE MILITARY

The military, one of the world's largest employers of nurses, discriminates on the basis of sexual orientation. Since 1993, the military has followed a policy of "don't ask, don't tell." Unlike the previous code, which banned all gay men and lesbians in the armed services, the new policy allows people to serve if they hide their sexual orientation, do not engage in same-gender sexual activity, and do not display affection for people of the same gender. The change was intended to prevent witch-hunts and put an end to unwarranted discharges. It has done neither.

The military discharges proportionately more lesbians than gay men. According to a General Accounting Office report in 1992, lesbians in all branches of the armed services combined are discharged at a rate two or three times higher than would be expected by the number of women in the military. The rate is almost six times higher in the Marine Corps (Cammermeyer, 1994).

The military came under fire in 1995, when a federal judge in Brooklyn ruled that the "don't ask, don't tell" policy was unconstitutional because it violates free-speech and equal-protection rights. According to *The Wall Street Journal* (McMorris, 1995), Army lawyers argued that openly lesbian and gay soldiers "will erode morale and undermine military readiness because heterosexual soldiers are opposed to serving alongside homosexuals."

Judge Nickerson did not agree that the military's reasons justify discrimination. Because the policy treats soldiers differently on the basis of sexual orientation, it violates equal-protection rights. The case was appealed to the Supreme Court but was not yet decided by press time.

Colonel Margarethe Cammermeyer

On April 28, 1989, Colonel Margarethe Cammermeyer started a chain reaction that changed public opinion about lesbians, nurses, and the injustice of discrimination in the military. During a screening interview for a top-secret clearance, she admitted, "I am a lesbian." Because her interview occurred before the military began its policy of "don't ask, don't tell, don't pursue," Cammermeyer's admission led to her discharge, a lengthy court battle, and a deep exploration of herself as a lesbian and a member of a community.

Her credentials were impeccable. She started in the Army Student Nurse Program in 1963 and soon served in Vietnam, where she was awarded the Bronze Star. She married, moved to suburban Seattle, and had four sons. In 1972, she joined the Army Reserves and steadily worked up the ranks to colonel and served as the state Chief Nurse of the Washington State National Guard. She also worked in Veteran Administration hospitals and in 1985 was honored as the VA's Nurse of the Year from a field of 34,000 nurses and received a letter of congratulations from President Reagan.

In 1989, she set her sights on becoming the nationwide Chief Nurse of the National Guard (one of only three national chief nurse positions), but first she needed to attend the Army's War College, which hinged on a top-secret security clearance. Why would someone so intelligent, dedicated, and hard-working risk everything by admitting she is a lesbian?

In her 1994 autobiography, *Serving in Silence*, Cammermeyer is portrayed at the time of her security interview as a forthright officer who trusted the military's integrity, but was inexperienced as a lesbian.

She met and eventually fell in love with her partner, Diane, only a year before her security interview. Admitting her sexual orientation was not the result of a carefully weighed risk-benefit analysis. Instead, it expressed the value she placed on service over personal attributes. She was unaware of the military's policy concerning homosexuals and had not known a gay or lesbian soldier who had suffered as a result of it. She wrote: "I believed the Constitution I had sworn to defend as a soldier permitted those, like myself, with unblemished records to serve regardless of the color of their skin, their ethnic background, their religion, or their sexual orientation."

Cammermeyer's real courage came during the long delays that plagued the military's investigation. She refused to retreat by resigning or retiring. After seven months, the Army declared its intention to discharge her; and in July 1991, a reluctant colonel recommended that she be discharged, although praising her leadership and outstanding accomplishments. After a second investigation by the Army, she was honorably discharged on June 11, 1992. Until the end, she served with unwavering professional commitment.

During the intervening three years, Cammermeyer worked with the Lambda Legal Defense and Education Fund and the Northwest Women's Law Center to prepare a civil suit following her inevitable discharge. The suit focused on prejudice. The military claimed that lesbians and gay men make discipline and morale impossible; and if they were allowed to serve, heterosexuals would understandably refuse to join the military or obey lesbian or gay officers. Despite strong evidence that out lesbians and gay men do not pose security risks, the military continued to cling to this unsubstantiated belief.

Because Cammermeyer was not involved in sexual misconduct and had a sterling record, her case demonstrated that the military's claims were based solely on prejudice. Finally in June 1994, Judge Thomas Zilly in Federal District Court in Seattle ruled that the miliary's policy was unconstitutional because it denied equal protection, " . . . the federal government cannot discriminate against a class in order to give effect to the prejudice of others." The court ordered that Cammermeyer be reinstated, and she again serves as the state Chief Nurse of the Washington National Guard. However, the military plans to appeal.

Cammermeyer does not urge other soldiers to come out. In *Serving in Silence* (1994), she wrote, "I always counsel them to stay silent, otherwise their careers would be annihilated" (p. 294). She refers them to the Military Law Task Force in San Diego or the Servicemembers Legal Defense Network in Washington, D.C.

Facing a Military Investigation

The policy of "don't ask, don't tell, don't pursue" changed the rules concerning gay and lesbian nurses in the military, but it has not eliminated the threat of harassment. According to the Servicemembers Legal Defense Network (SLDN) "Guidelines for Servicemembers and Civilian Friends Under 'Don't Ask, Don't Tell, Don't Pursue'" (undated):

> Military commanders and investigators, sometimes blatantly, and sometimes with the help of creative phrasing, continue to question recruits and servicemembers about their sexual orientation. They continue to launch investigations without credible evidence, and seize personal possessions, such as diaries, family letters, and photos of friends. Suspect servicemembers still face harassment, physical violence, jail, and an untimely end to their careers. Most servicemembers do not realize that the new policy affords little protection or privacy for lesbian and gay personnel, and most servicemembers do not know what their legal rights are under the new policy.

The SLDN offers legal advice and help for members of the armed services targeted by the military's policy on homosexuals through a nationwide network of over 200 attorneys. They also gather information and lobby to change policies that discriminate against gay and lesbian servicemembers.

Guidelines for Servicemembers

To protect yourself, the SLDN offers these guidelines if you are questioned about your private life or about your civilian friends:

Know Your Legal Rights

- ▾ Article 31 of the UCMJ gives military members the right to remain silent. Always consult with an attorney before giving up your rights.

- ▾ Investigators must stop all questioning and release you if you ask to consult with an attorney.

▾ Military investigators and inquiry officers have no juris-
diction over civilians.

Say Nothing

▾ Statements of sexual orientation or activities are still
grounds for discharge.

▾ If you want to stay in the military, anything you say can
and will be used against you. If you want to get out,
saying the wrong thing can ruin your discharge or get
you court-martialed.

▾ Doctors, psychologists, chaplains, legal officers, legal
assistants, and friends often do not keep secrets. What
you tell them may end up on your commander's desk.
Only a defense lawyer who represents you can be
counted on to keep information confidential.

▾ Civilians, including family members and friends, do not
have to speak with military officials, no matter what
they say. Civilians are permitted by law to record investigator's badge numbers and units and to refuse to
speak with them further. Military officials must stop all
attempts at questioning a civilian and leave the
premises, if asked to do so. Even the most innocent
statements can be used against a servicemember.

Sign Nothing   Even initials can waive your legal rights.

Get Legal Help   The new regulations are tricky—don't go it
alone. Organizations that provide confidential help include:
SLDN, 202-328-FAIR and the Military Law Task Force,
619-233-1701.

(These guidelines are written for military members who are
questioned about their private lives and their civilian friends.
Military members who are questioned about the private lives of
other servicemembers are not included in these guidelines and
should call the preceding phone numbers for appropriate counseling in this situation.)

Reprinted with permission of the Servicemembers Legal
Defense Network, P.O. Box 53013, Washington, D.C., 20009.

U.S. SUPREME COURT

The Supreme Court has ignored most cases contesting discrimination on the basis of sexual orientation. One notable exception is the criminal case of Bowers v. Hardwick.

In August 1982, a police officer arrested 28-year-old Michael Hardwick in the bedroom of his Atlanta home for having oral sex with another man. Both men were adults, acting in private, and consented to sex. Oral sex and anal sex are illegal—regardless of the gender of the people involved—under Georgia's 1816 sodomy law. Hardwick questioned the constitutionality of the state law. The Court of Appeals held that " . . . the Georgia statute violated respondent's fundamental rights because his homosexual activity is a private and intimate association that is beyond the reach of state regulation by reason of the Ninth Amendment and the due process clause of the Fourteenth Amendment."

In a close vote, the U.S. Supreme Court reversed the ruling of the Court of Appeals—Hardwick lost. Five out of nine justices were unimpressed by the issues of privacy and due process. Instead, they concentrated on the gender of the people involved and the authority of the state to regulate sex. Chief Justice Burger wrote " . . . there is no such thing as a fundamental right to commit homosexual sodomy . . . . This is essentially not a question of personal 'preference' but rather of the legislative authority of the State."

However, four justices disagreed. In the dissenting opinion, Justice Blackman wrote:

> The fact that individuals define themselves in a significant way through their intimate sexual relationships with others suggests, in a nation as diverse as ours, that there may be many 'right' ways of conducting those relationships, and that much of the richness of a relationship will come from the freedom an individual has to choose the form and nature of these intensely personal bonds.

He also criticized the Court's interpretation of privacy in the case. "Indeed, the right of an individual to conduct intimate relationships in the intimacy of his or her own home seems to me to be the heart of the Constitution's protection of privacy." (For a complete transcript of this decision, see Rubenstein, 1993.)

Current Challenges

Two lower court decisions—one outlawing state and local discrimination, and another supporting discrimination—are being appealed in the U.S. Supreme Court. In February 1995, the high court agreed to hear a complicated Colorado case. In a tug of war at the polls and in the state's courtrooms, civil rights for lesbians and gay men were approved, then banned, then the ban was challenged on constitutional grounds.[1]

In 1992, Colorado voters passed a state constitutional amendment that made it illegal for local governments or state policies to provide protection from discrimination based on sexual orientation. A suit prevented the must-discriminate amendment from going into effect. The state Supreme Court upheld the lower court's decision because the amendment violated the "equal protection" guarantee in the U.S. Constitution. The State of Colorado appealed to the U.S. Supreme Court. At issue was the notion of "special rights." According to *The Wall Street Journal* (Barrett, 1995), the state Supreme Court viewed the amendment " . . . as a violation of the 'fundamental right' of 'an independently identifiable group'—gay and bisexual citizens—'to participate equally in the political process.'" The state, on the other hand, argued that the amendment tried to " . . . preclude official state 'approval of homosexuality as a legitimate alternative lifestyle.'" And it " . . . was intended to prevent homosexuals and bisexuals from receiving preferred legal status . . . ."

The case is important because the tactics and rhetoric used in Colorado are being planned across the country to endorse

---

[1]On May 20, 1996 (just before press time), the Supreme Court ruled 60 to 3 that Colorado's 1992 Amendment 2 was unconstitutional. The court took a middle-of-the-road approach that protects existing local and state provisions prohibiting discrimination on the basis of sexual orientation, but the decision stopped short of identifying gay men and lesbians as a class of people deserving protection in the same fashion as members of racial minorities. Although the court's decision will have no immediate effect on serving in the military or same-gender marriages, the long-range implications are difficult to predict.

bigotry. In 1994, anti-gay and lesbian campaigns were attempted in ten other states (Barrett, 1995). In November 1995, voters considered statewide anti-lesbian and gay proposals in at least two states: Washington and Maine (Olson, 1995).

Considering a similar issue, a federal appeals court came to an entirely different decision. In May 1995, an anti-gay and lesbian referendum in Cincinnati was upheld by the 6th U.S. Circuit Court of Appeals, stating that sexual orientation is not "an identifiable class" (Federal, 1995). In 1993, voters reversed a previous policy of protecting gays and lesbians from discrimination and amended the city charter to forbid future protection (Olson, 1995). The Cincinnati case was appealed to the U.S. Supreme Court, and the case was undecided at press time.

STATE PROTECTION

Only eight states—California, Connecticut, Hawaii, Massachusetts, Minnesota, New Jersey, Vermont, and Wisconsin—prevent discriminatory employment practices on the basis of sexual orientation. In 18 states, executive orders offer some kind of protection. In the remaining states, discrimination is legal (National Gay & Lesbian Task Force, 1994).

Because state governments are large employers, their union contracts and personnel policies may offer protection. Even different departments within the same state government may offer different protections.

Child Custody

Many lesbian and gay parents conceal their sexual orientation because they fear losing custody of their children. Only 11 states have laws that make the parent's sexual orientation immaterial to custody arguments. In 11 other states, the courts have ruled that the parent's sexual orientation is a sufficient reason; and 17 additional states have decided that it may be a reason to deny custody, if the parent's sexual orientation adversely affects the child (Singer & Deschamps, 1994).

Adoption and foster parent regulations may also exclude gay men and lesbians. In 1995, two states forbade adoption or foster placement, and 11 other states were considering similar regulations. "Social science research has overwhelmingly demonstrated that sexual orientation has no relevance to an individual's ability to parent," said Kate Kendall, legal director of the National Center for Lesbian Rights, "and that lesbian and gay parents are as capable and committed as heterosexual parents" (National Center for Lesbian Rights, 1995).

Sharon Kowalski and Karen Thompson

One of the most celebrated custody battles involved adults. On November 13, 1983, a drunk driver hit Sharon Kowalski resulting in a closed head injury with severe neurological damage. In a coma, Sharon was incapable of making decisions about her care or communicating her wishes. She was not expected to live, but she started responding when her lover, Karen Thompson, visited.

The couple had lived together and in a private ceremony had exchanged rings as a symbol of their love and commitment. But they never came out to their friends or families, and they never documented their commitment through a durable power of attorney. Because they remained closeted, Sharon's parents were suddenly confronted with their daughter's sexual orientation during the crisis of a life-threatening injury.

The accident started an eight-year court battle between Sharon's parents and her lover over guardianship. Based on directions from Sharon's parents, nurses prohibited Karen from visiting. Without her lover, Sharon's recovery suffered dramatically. Karen wanted to take care of Sharon and ensure that she received comprehensive rehabilitation, but Sharon's parents disagreed with Karen about how best to care for Sharon. She was ultimately transferred to a custodial care facility and Karen was barred from visiting.

Instead of caving in to institutional bigotry, Karen fought back. She formed an alliance with the disabled community to expose the injustice. Because Sharon and Karen were closeted, Karen had difficulty proving the strength of their relationship in court. After eight years, the Minnesota Court of Appeals reversed a lower court ruling prohibiting Karen from being granted guardianship. This allowed Sharon to finally come home with Karen as her primary caretaker.

No one will ever know how much Sharon's recovery was stunted because she was separated from her lover during a crucial period of rehabilitation. It shows the health implications of institutional bigotry. The nurses who cooperated with the parents' directions to separate the lovers damaged their patient's health.

Sharon's story also illustrates the importance of coming out and putting decisions in writing. "We need to make it legally clear what we want, because the legal system doesn't acknowledge our relationships," says a lesbian nurse. "The health care and legal systems express their heterosexism. We need to protect ourselves, because our wishes can so easily be taken away."

State Sodomy Laws

At one time all states prohibited sodomy—oral sex, anal sex, and sex with animals. By 1995, there were still 21 states with sodomy laws. In 15 of the remaining states, sodomy laws apply regardless of sexual orientation, and six states refer only to same-sex couples (American Civil Liberties Union, undated).

The case of Bowers v. Hardwick heard by the Supreme Court demonstrates the power of sodomy laws to control, harass, and punish gay men and lesbians. Although sex is a small part of life, sodomy laws are used to justify discrimination in all aspects of life, including relationships, housing, child custody, and work-related issues.

State Boards of Nursing

In some states, lesbian and gay nurses risk losing their licenses. Because sodomy may be a felony, nurses convicted of a felony may lose their licenses. In some states, just being charged with a felony is sufficient reason to suspend a nurse's license until the charge is cleared. Approximately 5% of registered nurses are disciplined due to criminal convictions (Elliott & Heines, 1987). It is uncertain how many times sodomy is used as a weapon, but sodomy laws make gay and lesbian nurses unfairly vulnerable to hatemongers.

Lesbian and gay nurses are also vulnerable in states that require good moral character in order to be licensed. In a 1992 survey of its members, the National Council of State Boards of Nursing (1992) reported that 24 states still require good moral character.

Undoubtedly, the standards are sometimes unfairly applied to gay men and lesbians. One nurse remembers an incident involving a former classmate, "A gay male student was arrested for a trumped-up morals charge that he chose to fight. And there was a question if he could be licensed. He needed to get letters of support from nursing instructors, and a few were very reluctant to give their support."

LOCAL PROTECTION

According to the National Gay and Lesbian Task Force's report in February 1994, at least 127 cities, counties, or other municipalities offered some form of protection from discrimination based on sexual orientation. The least comprehensive form of protection is through mayoral or council proclamation banning discrimination for public employment. This form of protection exists in 39 cities or counties.

An additional 87 cities or counties have human rights ordinances that include lesbians and gay men. The most comprehensive ordinances cover public employment, public accommodations, private employment, education, housing, credit, and union practices. Only 26 cities or counties offer the most comprehensive protection.

Civil rights ordinances do not cover registration or benefits for domestic partners. As of 1993, only 13 municipal governments offered health insurance benefits for same-sex domestic partners, and only 25 municipalities recognized some form of same-sex domestic partnership (Singer & Deschamps, 1994).

PROTECTION THROUGH LABOR CONTRACTS

Labor contracts can ensure a formalized mechanism to grieve discrimination, but the specific words "on the basis of sexual orientation" must be included (Frank & Holcomb, 1990). The American Nurses Association (ANA) supports the inclusion of sexual orientation in contracts negotiated by state nurses associations. Contracts that include the standards of ANA's ethical code also protect gay and lesbian patients from discrimination by nurses. In addition, contracts can be used to negotiate benefits for domestic partners (see Chapter 5 for more information). When anti-discrimination language exists, the union steward may be your greatest ally.

Bill Fought Back

Even when discrimination based on sexual orientation is not outlawed, you may still be able to grieve if you are part of the civil service system. Bill was denied a promotion mainly because he is openly gay. Instead of knuckling under to prejudice, he filed a grievance and persevered through four hearings in ten months until a state hearings officer, a lawyer, decided in his favor.

The merit system identifies rules. In Bill's case, his boss failed to obey the proper recruitment rules and denied his promotion because of "non-merit factors." These factors, according to the state report, were "a continuing pattern of discrimination based on his sexual orientation and related outside activities."

Bill was prevented from discussing AIDS with school administrators because he was openly gay. This was considered specific evidence of a "discriminatory environment." The report stated: "That decision was no less discriminatory than a decision to deny a person with a disability, or an Hispanic person, the assignment of making a 'diversity' presentation because he or she is 'openly disabled' or 'openly Hispanic.'"

The outside activities that allegedly created conflicts of interest were associations to gay community organizations. The hearing officer concluded:

In essence, then, the Division's position amounts to a discriminatory and unfounded assumption that the Grievant's (Bill's) affiliation with gay organizations would produce a conflict of interest which justified denying him the position . . . . Put another way, the Division's conduct assumed that gay persons were incapable of reconciling the Division's AIDS policy positions with their own personal beliefs and activities.

Although Bill won, it was an exhausting battle that exacted a heavy personal toll. He remembers, "I questioned whether it was really worth it, or did I just imagine the discrimination. You feel that everybody is against you. The system is designed to convince you to give up."

Bill urges other nurses to fight discrimination. "It's far better for you emotionally, it's far better for your coworkers, and it's far better for your profession to be open about who you are. The system won't change unless you challenge it." As a result of his grievance, Bill's department has a policy of nondiscrimination on the basis of sexual orientation.

SUMMARY

Lesbian and gay nurses cannot take for granted that laws and employment rules work to protect their rights. Protect yourself by learning the details of your state and local civil rights statutes. Does your employer have a policy of preventing discrimination based on sexual orientation? How does your union represent the needs of gay people? Do not be afraid to use your employer's grievance procedure.

If you are targeted at work, keep a written journal detailing events, dates, names, and conversations. Follow your employer's grievance procedure carefully and begin the process early, before you are fired or demoted. Seek professional advice. Your local gay and lesbian community center can refer you to a lawyer with specific experience defending lesbian and gay people. The following national organizations may offer additional help or information.

American Civil Liberties Union
Lesbian and Gay Rights Project
132 West 43rd Street
New York, NY 10036
(check for local chapters)

Lambda Legal Defense & Education Fund
666 Broadway
New York, NY 10012
212-995-8585

National Center for Lesbian Rights
870 Market Street, Suite 570
San Francisco, CA 94102-3012
415-392-6257

National Gay & Lesbian Task Force
1517 U. Street, N.W.
Washington, D.C. 20009
202-332-6483

Servicemembers Legal Defense Network
P.O. Box 53013
Washington, D.C., 20009
202-328-FAIR

Military Law Task Force
1168 Union Street, Suite 201
San Diego, CA 92101
619-233-1701

References

American Civil Liberties Union. (undated). *Briefing paper: Lesbian and gay rights.* New York: Author.

Barrett, P. M. (1995, February 22). High court to decide whether states may ban laws protecting homosexuals. *The Wall Street Journal,* p. A10.

Cammermeyer, M. (1994). *Serving in silence.* New York: Viking.

Elliott, R. L., & Heines, M. J. (1987). *Disciplinary data bank: A longitudinal study.* Chicago: National Council of State Boards of Nursing.

Federal appeals court reverses ruling on gays. (1995, May 15). *The Wall Street Journal,* p. B10.

Frank, M., & Holcomb, D. (1990). *Pride at work: Organizing for lesbian and gay rights in unions.* New York: The Lesbian and Gay Labor Network.

McMorris, F. A. (1995, March 31). Judge rejects Clinton's policy on homosexuals in the military. *The Wall Street Journal,* p. B5.

National Center for Lesbian Rights. (1995, Spring). The homefront battle: The radical right's assault on lesbian and gay families. *NCLR Newsletter, 1,* 10.

National Council of State Boards of Nursing. (1992). *Profiles of member board: 1992.* Chicago: Author.

National Gay & Lesbian Task Force. (1994). *Lesbian, gay, and bisexual civil rights in the U.S.* Washington, DC: Author.

Olson, D. (1995, May 18). Appeals court upholds anti-gay initiatives. *Windy City Times,* pp. 1, 10, 20.

Rubenstein, W. B. (Ed.). (1993). *Lesbians, gay men, and the law.* New York: The New Press.

Servicemembers Legal Defense Network (undated). "Guidelines for Servicemembers and Civilian Friends Under 'Don't Ask, Don't Tell, Don't Pursue.'" Washington, DC.

Singer, B. L., & Deschamps, D. (1994). *Gay and lesbian stats: A pocket guide of facts and figures.* New York: The New Press.

5 | DOMESTIC PARTNERS AND BENEFITS

I wear a wedding ring, but I have to tell them it's my grandmother's. Inside I hate staying in the closet. It's like turning your back on your own. But coming out could endanger my staying in school.

A lesbian student

NO BENEFITS MEANS DISCRIMINATION

Outside of individual acts of discrimination, gay and lesbian nurses see the lack of acknowledgment of their committed relationships as the most obvious form of bigotry. If marriage is considered the most important decision heterosexuals can make, why is a relationship of equally strong commitment considered trivial or invisible for lesbian and gay people?

Heterosexual married partners enjoy a variety of benefits that are often not available to same-sex domestic partners, including health, dental, vision, and life insurance; bereavement leave; Social Security and pension benefits for survivors; unpaid leave of absence to care for an ill spouse or child. The federal

Family and Medical Leave Act mandates unpaid leave of absence to care for an ill spouse or child, but it does not extend protection to same-sex domestic partners.

Denying benefits for same-sex partners also creates an economic injustice, and forces lesbian and gay nurses to underwrite the benefits of heterosexual families. This chapter examines the nature of gay and lesbian relationships and gives examples of employers offering benefits for domestic partners.

NAMING COMMITTED RELATIONSHIPS

What word best describes people of the same gender in a loving, committed relationship? *Friend* or *roommate*, the code words of the Cold War generation, are obviously too casual and do not convey the sense of mutual responsibility and commitment. *Lover*, the word frequently used by the hippie generation, is for many people too confrontational and overemphasizes the sexual aspects of a relationship. *Partner*, or its policy manual cousins, *spousal equivalent, same-sex domestic partner,* or *significant other* come closer to reflecting the serious nature of the relationship, but sound too formal. A stranger might assume it is just a business relationship without much affection.

Today, some people use traditional words to describe traditional relationships: two *husbands* or two *wives* are *married* to one another. Or if they wish to be a little less out, *spouse* may be the best word. *Girlfriend* and *boyfriend* emphasize companionship, rather than commitment, or are used when the relationship is new. These terms were used most often by the youngest people interviewed, regardless of the depth of their relationship.

Others would argue that many lesbians and gay men share committed, mutually supportive, loving relationships, but choose not to live under the same roof. They could be *partners* but not *domestic partners*. Many people struggle to adapt language to describe the true nature of their relationship, rather than restrict themselves to the narrow confines of the traditional forms that have names.

DISCRIMINATION AGAINST PARTNERS

Regardless of the words used to describe gay and lesbian families, some heterosexual nurses know that they are against them. In response to plans by the magazine *California Nursing* in 1991 to feature an article about gay and lesbian nurses, a nurse wrote in part the following letter to the editor:

> I do not believe that homosexual couples should be represented in the same way as married couples. Strong traditional families have been the bedrock of Western society. They bring children into the world and nurture them to adulthood. Homosexual "domestic partnerships" are transitory, do not reproduce, and do not train others in sound morals (Masulis, 1991). (From *California Nursing*. Reprinted with permission of the publisher.)

Fortunately, the editor ran the article based on an editorial policy "to give voice to all California nurses." She also asked in print: "If nurses cannot acknowledge or accept gay or lesbian colleagues, how can they deliver unbiased, non-judgmental care to gay and lesbian patients or to any minority?" (Stephany, 1991) (From *California Nursing*. Reprinted with permission of the publisher.)

More importantly, a growing number of voters favor local ordinances supporting same-sex domestic partners; and hospitals and universities are beginning to extend benefits to domestic partners.

HOW MANY IN COMMITTED RELATIONSHIPS?

It is impossible to know the exact number of gay and lesbian people in relationships, or how many live together. Because of discrimination, many lesbian and gay people lie on census or survey forms, and keep their relationships a secret. However, a

1992 survey found that 55.5% of gay men and 71.2% of lesbians were in steady relationships (Singer & Deschamps, 1994).

A 1988 study of gay and lesbian couples revealed that the couples had been together an average of six years, and 80% of the couples had been together more than a year. Most of the couples, 87% of the women and 93% of the men, lived together (Singer & Deschamps, 1994).

Of the 108 nurses interviewed for this book, 39% said that they lived with a partner, ranging from honeymoon to over 20 years.

GAY AND LESBIAN PARENTS

A few of the men and 30% of the women interviewed for this book are raising children, usually their biological children or their partner's offspring. Nationwide, an estimated 1 to 5 million lesbians are mothers and 1 to 3 million gay men are fathers. Between 6 and 14 million U.S. children have a gay or lesbian parent. Approximately 10,000 are the children of lesbians who were artificially inseminated (Singer & Deschamps, 1994).

Almost all of the children of the nurses interviewed for this book were born during a previous heterosexual marriage. After coming out, many of the nurses did not hide their sexual orientation from their former spouses. Some nurses even continued to share parenting responsibilities with their former spouses.

But a few nurses have to hide. "I can't admit that I'm a lesbian to my ex-husband, because it could be used in a custody battle," says a nurse in the South. "I could have my son taken away. I just can't trust him." An increasing number of states either ban lesbians and gay men from adopting or having custody of their own children.

Coming Out to Children

All of the nurses have either already come out to their children or plan to when the child reaches the right age. Explains one nurse, "When my daughter was around 11, she asked why people say (*offensive slang for gay man*). I told her it was because of prejudice. She knew what was going on emotionally between me and my lover, but she didn't have a word for it. When I told her I was gay, she didn't have a lot of questions. It wasn't very dramatic."

Some children dealt with anger due to loss when their parents divorced from a heterosexual marriage, and one parent also came out. Teenagers seem especially vulnerable. According to one nurse, "My marriage broke up at the same time I was coming out. The kids had huge problems with losing their father, and perhaps also questioning their own sexuality. It had much more to do with the divorce, than with my sexual orientation. They tried to come around very fast, but they were angry."

Another nurse discussed how discrimination affected her young daughter. "She lost her best friend. Because I was gay, they couldn't be friends. I confronted the mother, who was concerned that I would molest her daughter, and that being a lesbian was contagious. It didn't matter who I was, she went by what the Bible said."

Although most of the lesbian and gay parents interviewed for this book worried that their children might have a hard time dealing with their parent's sexual orientation, none of the children had long-lasting problems. Dozens of studies during the last 15 years confirm that children raised in gay and lesbian families are as well adjusted and happy as children from heterosexual families. The children develop the same and are no more likely than other children to become gay (Singer & Deschamps, 1994).

Sharing the Responsibilities of Parenting

Nurses with domestic partners share parenting responsibilities with their partner. Some of the nurses talked about the challenges of merging childrearing styles within the same household, when both partners have children of their own. "I became less of Attila-the-Hun mom, and my lover became less warm-and-fuzzy mom. Together we found a way that worked."

Another nurse talked about the impact on her son when her relationship ended. "I broke up with a lover of long standing when my son was a teenager. He was very angry at me. But his school counselor said it was like a divorce, not because I was a lesbian."

HOW RELATIONSHIPS GROW

Gay men and lesbians in relationships, just as heterosexual couples, change as the relationship grows and lengthens. Not every couple grows in exactly the same way, but researchers have described a pattern of growth. Couples move through stages at different rates, start at different places, stop or rest at different places, or return to an earlier stage to suit their individual needs. Stages are a way to describe people, not to pigeonhole or judge them.

Gay Men

By interviewing 156 long-term gay male couples, McWhirter and Mattison (1984) found six stages of development.

Blending   Similar to the honeymoon phase of heterosexual relationships, men in the first year want to do everything together. They delight in each other's company, the willing captives of love. They make love frequently, passionately, and only with each other.

Nesting   During the next one or two years, gay men make a home together and work out the chores of homemaking. Gay men seldom divide the chores into male and female stereotypes.

Maintaining   For the next couple of years, men return to developing their individual interests and pursuits. By this time, men trust one another more than they did when their relationship began, so they can risk being more assertive and worry less if their actions create conflict. While they explore individual interests, they also build traditions as a couple.

Building   While continuing to explore their separate interests, men in this stage deepen the strength of their life together. They rely and depend on each other.

Releasing   Between 11 and 20 years together, men may take each other for granted, but they trust each other more, and merge their finances and possessions.

Renewing After more than 20 years in a relationship, men restore a closeness in their relationship that is based on the security of having weathered years together through both good and bad times.

Lesbians

Doctors D. Merilee Clunis and G. Dorsey Green (1993), psychologists in private practice, also described six stages for lesbians in relationships.

Prerelationship Similar to "dating" in heterosexual relationships, women in this stage get to know one another. Each asks herself: Who is this woman? Does she want a relationship? Is this relationship worth exploring? Does her idea of a relationship match mine?

Romance Women in this stage burn with passion and feel perfectly accepted, understood, and appreciated. Because women strive for intimacy, lesbian honeymoons are intense.

Conflict Eventually reality sets in. No one could be as perfect as her lover first assumed. If the relationship survives, and many do, the partners learn how to deal with conflict, make mutual decisions, and arrive at shared goals for their relationship.

Acceptance Out of conflict comes a deeper affection and respect, without denying the partner's shortcomings or forgetting her strengths.

Commitment Women trust each other, and put temporary conflicts in the perspective of a long-term relationship. They work at ways of meeting or balancing their individual needs, while reinforcing the strength of their relationship together.

Collaboration After learning that conflict does not spell the end of relationship, women use the security of their relationship to build a bridge to a bigger world. They may decide to start a joint business, raise children, or work for social or political causes.

COMPARING RELATIONSHIPS

Compared to heterosexual relationships, gay men and lesbian couples may move in together sooner, but they merge their finances much later. Many do not have a joint checking account or own property jointly until they have lived together for several years.

Unlike heterosexual marriages, which begin with a grand and well-planned ceremony, lesbians and gay men usually do not announce the beginning of their relationship. Frequently, co-workers and family members find out after the fact. If they ultimately have a ceremony to celebrate their love, it usually happens after they have lived together for a couple of years.

Entering a relationship may also force the merging of two very different styles of being out. Just sharing a household with another person of the same gender is a form of coming out that may create conflict.

Being in a relationship can heighten the injustice of discrimination. Parents who would welcome a son's wife or a daughter's husband may scorn his husband or her wife. Coworkers who understand the desire to share holidays and special occasions with their family, may expect gay men and lesbians to volunteer to work holidays because they do not have a real "family."

GAY AND LESBIAN RELATIONSHIPS

Dr. Letitia Peplau (1991), a social psychologist and researcher, provided an extensive summary of research findings about lesbian and gay relationships.

- ▾ Gay and lesbian couples express love and commitment in diverse ways.
- ▾ Most lesbians and gay men value committed, long-lasting relationships. A slightly higher proportion of lesbians than gay men are in relationships.

▾ As with heterosexual marriages, same-sex relationships of 20 years or longer are not uncommon. But research does not show that lesbian relationships necessarily last longer than gay men's relationships.

▾ Gay men and lesbians love their partners and are satisfied with their relationships.

▾ Most lesbian and gay couples do not follow traditional "husband" and "wife" roles in their relationships. Instead, most gay men and lesbians have a "peer" or "friendship" form of relationship. Both partners share similar interests, share power and resources equally, and make important decisions collaboratively. Chores or tasks within the relationship are usually determined by personal interest or skill. Both partners usually work.

▾ Same-sex couples usually have a circle of people they can draw on for emotional and material support. But they rely more on friends than on family members for help. Couples with children, however, are more likely to turn to their families for support.

▾ Relationships are influenced more by gender than by sexual orientation.

▾ Gay male couples have the highest frequency of sexual activity, followed by heterosexual couples, followed by lesbian couples. All three kinds of couples are equally satisfied with their sex lives, and the frequency of sexual activity decreases as time goes on. Sexual fidelity is less common among gay men.

▾ Lesbian and gay relationships are not any more dysfunctional than are heterosexual relationships. Although gay and lesbian couples face unique problems caused by discrimination, their relationships are no more troubled than are heterosexual relationships.

▾ Studying lesbian and gay couples helps researchers learn more about all couples including heterosexual couples.

SANCTIONS FOR RELATIONSHIPS

Marriage is still illegal for same-sex partners in all of the states in the United States. As of September 1993, however, 25 cities, townships, and counties recognized domestic partners in some fashion (Singer & Deschamps, 1994).

Several churches sanctify committed same-sex relationships through ceremonies. Partners attest their love and commitment and receive the clergy's blessing before a community of friends and family. Many partners also exchange rings. Some wear their rings on the left hand as a symbol of the tradition of marriage, and others use the right hand to signify a relationship that is deep but significantly different than heterosexual marriages.

HOSPITALS OFFERING BENEFITS

On January 1, 1995, the University of Michigan, which includes the University of Michigan Medical Center, began offering health insurance, dental insurance, and dependent group life insurance for same-sex domestic partners. The university limits the benefit to same-sex partners because opposite-sex partners can marry and receive benefits. To qualify, a domestic partner:

1. is the same sex as the faculty, staff member, or student, and

2. is not legally married to another individual, and

3. is not related to the faculty, staff member, or student by blood in a manner that would bar marriage, and

4. is registered either publicly or privately as a Domestic Partner with a municipality offering formal registration, and

5. has allowed at least six months to pass since a statement of termination of a previous same-sex domestic partnership.

The university also stipulates that: "Children of a same-sex domestic partner who are in the custody and care of and legally dependent on the same-sex domestic partner and are members of the household of the faculty, staff member, or student are also eligible for the benefit plans."

Registering Same-Sex Domestic Partners

The university's policy concerning same-sex domestic partners reflects the liberal attitudes of Ann Arbor, where the university is located. Ann Arbor voters approved a Domestic Partnership Ordinance in 1991. The city clerk records domestic partnership, but the documents can be registered or kept in private. Appendix A reprints the information sheet sent by the City of Ann Arbor to explain domestic partnership.

The University of Pennsylvania Health Systems

In 1995, the University of Pennsylvania Health Systems (UPHS) also began offering benefits for same-sex domestic partners. Unlike the University of Michigan, the UPHS is an employer separate from the university. Because no local ordinance sanctions domestic partnership, employees must register their relationships directly with the UPHS. Children are covered if they are registered on the UPHS's Certification of Domestic Partnership with supporting documentation, such as a birth certificate or adoption decree.

ORGANIZING BENEFITS

The struggle for benefits for same-sex domestic partners is different with each employer. It seems to be easier in cities that endorse domestic partnerships, and where either local ordinances or an employer's policies prevent discrimination on the basis of sexual orientation. Although universities are often considered liberal, and may be expected to extend benefits, the same universities may be burdened with powerful and conservative alumni associations, or fear that the publicity would risk their funding from other sources.

Some hospitals offer benefits for same-sex domestic partners because an administrator pushed the issue. A nurse explains, "A gay man is in charge of the benefits section at our hospital. No group got together, but several people provided steady, gentle pressure."

Collective Bargaining

Labor unions sometimes negotiate for benefits for domestic partners. The Lesbian and Gay Labor Network (Frank & Holcomb, 1990) recommends starting to organize support a year before the contract expires. Form a committee on domestic partnership issues and make sure that other union committees dealing with family issues understand domestic partnership issues. Try to make allies on the pre-bargaining and negotiating committees. If your union formally surveys members to determine issues, convince your gay and lesbian colleagues and heterosexual allies to identify benefits for domestic partners as a priority issue. Strength comes from numbers. Unions may refuse to jeopardize their other issues by advocating for a risky position that is perceived to directly affect few members.

Expect that full benefits for domestic partners may take several contract rounds to achieve. Identify which benefits are inexpensive and easy to implement, such as bereavement leave, and which benefits are costly, such as health insurance and pension benefits. Try to put a realistic dollar value on presumed expensive benefits. Usually, fewer people than expected apply for benefits, and the cost is less than anticipated.

Influencing Benefits without Unions

At other hospitals, lesbian and gay employees have organized informally. One nurse described the process used at her hospital. "We presented the issue on moral grounds," she explains. "The hospital has an explicit policy not to discriminate on the basis of sexual orientation, so we told them now it's time to make that policy real by putting an end to discrimination in the way benefits are offered."

Ten gay and lesbian employees formed a committee headed by a fervent supporter. "You need a single person to take this on as his cause and call frequently to move it forward," she says.

The committee offered emotional support, as well as people to help with the grunt work.

The committee spent two months gathering signatures on a petition supporting benefits for same-sex domestic partners. About 200 employees (out of a total of approximately 5,000 employees) signed, and only one nurse refused to sign. Although the number was relatively small, it showed a broad base of support, and it suggested that a much larger number of signatures could be gathered if necessary.

The committee presented its requests to an influential administrator. Although he supported the idea, he was uncertain of the economics. Unseen by the committee, the hospital's legal department examined the hospital's interest, while the administrator conducted a cost analysis. Several months later, the legal department reported that the hospital did not have a legal obligation to extend benefits to same-sex domestic partners, but nothing prevented the benefits legally. The cost analysis showed that benefits would not have an unreasonable financial impact.

Nine months after the committee first met, the hospital announced benefits for same-sex domestic partners. "Whether or not this had a practical value, it had a validating effect on my relationship," says one organizer.

THE COST OF BENEFITS

The cost of benefits to the employer is usually small. According to the Lambda Legal Defense and Education Fund (undated), the cost to the City of Madison, Wisconsin, for health insurance for same-sex and opposite-sex domestic partners was estimated to increase the city's insurance premiums by only 1 to 3%.

The actual costs are frequently smaller than projected because few people register for benefits. For example, the City of San Francisco estimated that 2,000 employees would apply; but, according to the National Center for Lesbian Rights (1992), only 175 enrolled—36 lesbian couples, 56 gay male couples, and 83 heterosexual couples.

At Levi Strauss & Company, out of approximately 25,000 employees, only 250 enrolled; and the company estimates that 40 to 45% of those enrolled are in same-sex couples (Lambda,

undated). The cost to Levi Strauss is expected to rise by only ½%
(National Center for Lesbian Rights, 1992).

At New York's Montefiore Medical Center, the university
hospital for the Albert Einstein College of Medicine, only two
dozen out of approximately 6,000 employees enrolled for benefits for same-sex domestic partners (Lambda, undated).

PENSION BENEFITS

In the 1994 election, voters in San Francisco passed a proposal
extending pension benefits to domestic partners of city workers.
Because Social Security benefits do not apply to surviving same-
sex domestic partners, employer pension programs are important
to lesbian and gay workers. To appreciate the San Francisco
proposition, first compare it to other plans currently in use.

Most hospitals have two systems of providing retirement
income for employees. Using the first method, employees con-
tribute to their own individual retirement account, and some hospitals match part or all of the contribution. This form of
retirement is already available to same-sex domestic partners, if
the employee designates the partner as the account's beneficiary.
Because the account always has a dollar value, based on the
amount contributed and market fluctuations, the surviving partner inherits the money.

The second kind of pension plan relies solely on the
employer's contributions. The employees' benefits depend on
salary and number of years of service. At retirement, the
employee receives a fixed amount each month for the remainder
of life. This kind of plan does not have an inheritable value, but
some plans continue to pay heterosexual spouses after the
employee dies. This is the most familiar kind of plan, and except
in San Francisco, it does not continue to pay same-sex domestic
partners after the employee dies.

OTHER BENEFITS

Without incurring a great expense, employers can extend
bereavement leave to survivors of domestic partnerships. Many

gay- and lesbian-friendly organizations already offer these benefits. The New York State Nurses Association negotiated bereavement leave at Mt. Sinai hospital for the death of "a person with whom the employee had a spouse-like relationship" (Frank & Holcomb, 1990).

Unpaid leave as described in the Family and Medical Leave Act could also be easily extended to domestic partners. Ironically, the act protects a woman's job if she needs unpaid leave in order to care for her brother with AIDS; but his lover's job security remains unprotected if he needs leave to care for the same man.

Some hospitals also allow nurses to use time from their sick time bank to care for their spouses or children when they are sick. This could easily be applied to anyone who resides within the same household, regardless of the title of the relationship.

SUMMARY

Gay and lesbian nurses know that their relationships are as strong and committed as heterosexual marriages. Researchers agree. Denying benefits to same-sex domestic partners is based on myths and misunderstanding about gay and lesbian relationships, and is a visible sign of discrimination. Yet many employers are capable of changing their policies when confronted with the ethical injustice of discrimination or the bargaining power of gay and lesbian employees. The economic cost of providing benefits for same-sex domestic partners is very small compared to the value of attracting and retaining highly skilled lesbian and gay professionals.

References

Clunis, D. M., & Green, G. D. (1993). *Lesbian couples: Creating healing relationships for the '90s.* Seattle: Seal Press.

Frank, M., & Holcomb, D. (1990). *Pride at work: Organizing for lesbian and gay rights in unions.* New York: Lesbian and Gay Labor Network.

Lambda Legal Defense & Education Fund. (undated). *Negotiating for equal employment benefits: Resource packet.* New York: Author.

Masulis, K. (1991). Gay/lesbian nurses [Letter to the editor]. *California Nursing, 13*(3), 35.

McWhirter, D., & Mattison, A. (1984). *The male couple: How relationships develop.* Englewood Cliffs, NJ: Prentice-Hall.

National Center for Lesbian Rights. (1992). *Recognizing lesbian and gay families: Strategies for obtaining domestic partners benefits.* San Francisco: Author.

Peplau, L. A. (1991). Lesbian and gay relationships. In J. Gonsiorek & J. Weinrich (Eds.), *Homosexuality: Research implications for public policy* (pp. 177–196). Newbury Park, CA: Sage.

Singer, B., & Deschamps, D. (Eds.). (1994). *Gay and lesbian stats: A pocket guide of facts and figures.* New York: The New Press.

Stephany, T. M. (1991). The invisible presence: Gay and lesbian nurses. *California Nursing, 13*(3), 20–22.

SPECIAL PROBLEMS: HIV DISEASE AND CHEMICAL DEPENDENCY

How can we appreciate that life is a gift? How can we use our time well? We can use this experience as a way to improve the quality of life. We try to help our patients do it all the time. We don't do it enough for ourselves.

A gay nurse infected with HIV

Being gay didn't cause me to be a user, but it sure helped . . . . Being a nurse also helped. I had free access to needles, and I developed excellent technique at giving IV injections. Being a nurse also prevented me from seeking treatment sooner—I thought a nurse couldn't be an addict.

A recovering gay nurse

MOST ARE DRUG-FREE AND UNINFECTED

Although the majority of gay and lesbian nurses are sober, drug-free, and not infected with HIV, these problems—chemical dependency and AIDS—need special consideration. Gay men are at increased risk of HIV infection, and gay men and lesbians share a higher risk for chemical dependency. These problems may heighten the stigma already faced by lesbian and gay nurses and may force the issue of whether or not to come out.

The vast majority of impaired nurses are heterosexual. But a greater percentage of gay men and lesbians—perhaps as much as three times the rate for the general public—have problems with chemical dependency or alcohol. Many experts, however, question these estimates because early researchers only sampled people who frequented lesbian or gay bars. This may have led to overestimates.

Although nurses use drugs for complex reasons, prejudice certainly contributes to their use. Stigma delays many nurses from seeking treatment, and prejudice or ignorance on the part of many therapists reduces the effectiveness of treatment.

HOW MANY ARE INFECTED?

Between 1 and 1.5 million Americans are infected with HIV. According to the CDC (as of October 31, 1995) 501,310 Americans have been diagnosed with AIDS, and 62% have died. Although women and heterosexuals are the fastest growing groups of people infected, gay and bisexual men are still the hardest hit. Roughly 86% of the people diagnosed with AIDS are men, 51% have had sex with other men, and an additional 7% are injection drug users and have had sex with men (CDC, 1995). AIDS has wiped out entire groups of friends, and left gaping holes in some gay communities across the country. As the epidemic continues, more and more people in small and medium-sized cities are affected.

Approximately 14% of people diagnosed with AIDS are women, usually infected through IV drug use or sex with IV drug users. About 7% of men and women with AIDS were infected though heterosexual contact, and 25% through IV drug use. Lesbians who use injection drugs are at risk for HIV infection.

NURSES WITH HIV DISEASE

No one knows exactly how many gay and lesbian nurses are infected with HIV. In April 1994, *RN* magazine reported that approximately 2,600 nurses had developed AIDS, and about half had died. More nurses have been infected than any other group of health care professionals. But few were infected at work. According to *RN*, only 13 nurses have documented work-related infections ("Latest CDC," 1994). Most of the nurses infected with HIV are gay men who became infected through their personal sexual and drug habits.

Women who have sex exclusively with other women are much less at risk. In a study of 18 long-term couples, where one partner was infected through injection drug use, the other women remained uninfected despite oral-genital sex, anal manipulation, or sex during menstruation (Raiteri, Fora, & Sinicco, 1994).

Injection drug users, regardless of their sexual orientation, remain at high risk of becoming infected. Ironically, lesbians share the stigma of AIDS in the popular imagination. In a survey of 278 nursing students concerning lesbians, 28% of the students felt that "Lesbians are a high risk group for AIDS" (Eliason, Donelan, & Randall, 1992).

PROFILES OF NURSES WITH HIV DISEASE

Several men agreed to talk about their HIV disease. All had become infected through sexual contact between five and ten years ago. One nurse adamantly decided to hide his diagnosis from his coworkers and employer. Others chose to share their diagnosis and received support. One man was forced to take a medical leave of absence because of rapidly worsening dementia. Several uninfected nurses reported that coworkers or friends had been fired or forced to work beyond their physical capability and were compelled to quit.

A nurse in the Midwest, who was assumed by her co-workers to be heterosexual, reports the way some nurses gossip about an HIV-infected coworker:

> Bob is HIV positive. When his performance falls below perfection, they cut him for being HIV positive. Or when his mood is off, they make little rude comments like, "He must need to get laid, but of course he can't." Or when he leaves his coffee cup out, they pick it up and ask "Where's the disinfectant?" At first it shocked me, they said so many cruel things. When it's time for him to change incontinent pads on male patients, they joke that it takes him so long because he's playing with their (*slang for penis*). They joke that it's the only chance he gets to play with one now that he's HIV positive. They all laugh.

Tasteless jokes behind a coworker's back are one form of prejudice. Other forms of discrimination include losing malpractice insurance or employment because of unfounded fears. Naphtali Offen, from the Gay and Lesbian Medical Society, formerly called the American Association of Physicians for Human Rights, has counseled hundreds of infected health care workers as part of the organization's medical expertise retention program. The program offers information, counseling, advocacy, and legal referrals for all HIV-infected health care professionals regardless of sexual orientation.

He cautions, "Think long and hard before you disclose your HIV infection at work even to your friends. Keep your mouth shut until you know the facts. Generally I think it's better for us all to be out, but I've seen too many people hurt because they trusted that their friends at work would do the right thing."

Even if the discriminating hospital is clearly wrong, it may take years to fight in court. Unfortunately, most infected nurses cannot afford the time it takes to mount a wrongful termination suit. Some infected nurses die before their case is decided.

Nurses infected with HIV often feel isolated. Disclosing HIV disease means coming out, and gay men and lesbians cannot yet count on support or freedom from discrimination. Even 15 years into the epidemic, many heterosexual nurses are fearful of becoming infected with HIV through casual contact. Nurses already frustrated by misunderstanding about lesbian and gay people may not want to deal with the additional misunder-standings surrounding AIDS. Some infected nurses also feel scorned because they are expected to answer to a higher standard—as nurses, they should have known how to avoid infection.

Bill Is Out

Bill is open about his HIV disease and uses his personal experiences when he talks about HIV and AIDS. He is out at work about being gay so he decided to come out about his HIV disease. "The way people deal with HIV disease is a microcosm of the way they deal with being gay," says Bill. "It's important to tell someone at work, so you can get support. Otherwise the isolation adds to the misery. Or if it's too risky at work, join a support group outside of work."

Bill first came out to his supervisor, then he announced it at a staff meeting. "It can be very scary to come out with HIV disease. I didn't know how my coworkers would respond. It was very emotional with hugging and kissing, but afterward no one even mentioned it to me. I didn't know if they were disinterested, or if they didn't know how to talk about it."

Through his experience, Bill has learned what it means to need, as well as give support. "Nurses are good at giving supportive initial responses, but poor at sustained support. Think of HIV disease as any other loss or emotional issue. HIV-negative nurses should stick their neck out and offer, 'What can I do for you?' or, 'I want you to know that I'm there for you.' In response, HIV-infected nurses need to be open and honest about their feelings and when they need help."

He reminds infected nurses to recognize when it is time to cut back to a part-time schedule or go on disability. "You don't have to wait until you're burned out and angry to leave. If you do AIDS work, give yourself permission to consider something else. If you decide to go on disability, have a plan about what you're going to do."

Bill is selective about talking about his HIV disease with patients. "I trust my intuition. I've told some patients, and didn't tell others. I wouldn't come out to a patient if I worked on a non-AIDS unit."

He also advises nurses to consult their doctor, if they are concerned about working on a particular unit because of the potential health risks. "If you're really conservative, then avoid patient contact. But most opportunistic infections are from your own body."

The basic questions for Bill extend beyond work: "How can we appreciate that life is a gift? How can we use our time well? We can use this experience as a way to improve our own quality of life. We try to help our patients do it all the time. We don't do it enough for ourselves."

Kevin's Experience

Kevin works as a case manager and educator for other people with HIV disease. Infected over 10 years ago, he remains symptom free except for very mild peripheral neuropathy. "I have a long history of being out as a gay man," he explains, "so sharing my HIV diagnosis is part of the pattern of my life."

As a result, Kevin gets more attention or mothering from his coworkers. "They pay more attention to my minor illnesses, and they caution me when I'm overextending," he says. His coworkers also ask about his T-cell counts. "You know you're going to be scrutinized. It's like I should post my results on the bulletin board because I'm going to be asked so many times."

Does he tell his clients that he too has HIV disease? "It's more complex disclosing your HIV disease to clients. For several years I didn't. Now I pick and choose. For some it creates a bond, but for others it would decrease my effectiveness as a case manager."

He sometimes questions how long he will continue to provide care for people with AIDS. "I go through periods where I grow tired of doing HIV work and losing clients. I don't want to sit around and talk about HIV all day. Day by day I want to go on and continue the work, but there is an accumulated stress. It helps to have loving friends and coworkers. I would have a far different attitude if I had to hide at work."

Harry Decided Not to Tell

Harry first knew he was infected with HIV seven years ago. He used the information to plan for his eventual retirement. "Always look at benefit packages and buy the best supplemental insurance you can afford, then don't quit. Strongly consider staying at a job you don't love."

"I wanted to save some good time for myself." But the first time he shared his HIV diagnosis with his coworkers or supervisor was when he gave his two-week notice of retirement. "I didn't want to screw the hospital, but I had to take care of myself."

Harry retired ten months ago with 70% of his gross salary and full medical and dental benefits. Combined with his benefits from supplemental disability insurance policies, he now earns more than he did when he worked. He spends time traveling, enjoying music and theater, and cementing relationships with his friends.

Recently, his vision has failed because of a viral infection and his doctors have been unable to definitively diagnose a lung mass. Each lung biopsy caused a pneumothorax. As he talks, sitting in the sun in the backyard tethered to a bulky infusion pump, his chest caves in during each inhalation. He points to a scar caused by a new device used to treat pneumothorax. He easily gets off the subject, in part because of mild dementia, in part because he needs a nap, in part because of profound anemia, and in part because he has so many interests. Later this afternoon, a volunteer will drop by to help; and tomorrow he will be transfused at home.

"What would you have to gain by revealing that you're infected that could possibly outweigh putting yourself at such grave risk? There are still pockets of ignorance. If you got fired or laid off, then what happens to your benefits? You could only gain a catharsis, and that's what a support system is for. If you tell, then who's in control? Not you. If you keep it to yourself, you stay in control."

Harry decided to retire because the hospital was planning to reduce benefits and lay people off. "I was getting nervous. I didn't want to risk getting laid off. When I told them, there were tears and hugs—it was just awful. I was comforting them. Most people knew I'm gay because I talked about gay things; and one or two said that they had guessed that I was sick. There was all this support afterward. They invited me to unit parties, and offered to help at home."

If you are planning to retire, Harry advises doing your homework first. "Line up professional advice and support, and get all your information before you make the move."

When asked if he missed nursing, he said, "You leave everything behind. I miss work, but not as much as I miss my sight or breathing. I miss contact with the children who were my patients, but not the crazy health factory."

Three months later, Harry died quietly at home. On autopsy, the lung mass was diagnosed as lymphoma.

George Denied His Problem

George never shared his diagnosis with his coworkers and supervisor, even when his HIV disease was severe. He always received good evaluations, no one ever questioned his competence, and he never called in sick. But it eventually became obvious that he was becoming more and more demented, and he was putting himself and his patients at risk. His nurse manager tells the story.

"I don't think that he would have chosen to work when his dementia made him dangerous, but he didn't have enough self-awareness to make that judgment."

In the beginning, George had subtle problems—trouble adding up I & Os or taking a half-hour to count the narcotics. But his coworkers covered for him. "Everyone suspected that he had AIDS because he was losing weight and wasting away. His usual personality also made it harder to get a handle on a possible problem. He was quirky. If the staff hadn't protected him as much, he could have gotten help sooner. But I had to wait until there was tangible evidence before I confronted him—you can't just guess."

The first opportunity to confront George came when he drew up an oral antacid into a 50 cc syringe for a patient with a central line. "He told me he wasn't going to take the port off. I made sure that he poured it into a med cup and gave it to the patient to drink. I also gave him an oral warning. But he denied that there was a bigger problem."

The second incident involved insulin. "I saw him use a 3 cc syringe to draw it up. I confronted him with his poor judgment, but he didn't understand why I was reprimanding him. It was OK that he was mad at me. I knew I was doing the right thing. The same day, I asked for his permission to talk with his doctor, who told me that George had requested not to receive any treatment." The doctor worked with the nurse manager to facilitate George going on a medical leave of absence.

Although the nurse manager had George's interests in mind, his director was not supportive. "My director initially wanted to have him suspended and fired because of his continued errors. But I couldn't fire him and still live with myself. I refused to give her George's name or his doctor's name in order to protect his confidentiality. I convinced her that a leave of absence was best." The same director later demanded to know the names of all the lesbian and gay staff. "I told her that I had no way to know, and I cared about nurses' performance not their sexual orientation."

George did not work again. The same day as the insulin incident, he went on a medical leave of absence to allow the nurse manager time to convince him to apply for disability. Soon after, he retired with 80% of his regular salary and full medical benefits. He went to live with his parents out of state, and regularly called his friends at work. Six months later he died.

George's illness and leave of absence were emotionally difficult for the staff. "Even the people who didn't like George felt ambivalent and sad for him. Some were angry at me and wondered if he was being trashed. They worried how he was going to survive. Nurses on his shift worried about who was going to take care of him. They frequently brought him food at work and watched out for him."

But others were relieved that the responsibility of covering for him and protecting him was finally lifted. They had been giving him a progressively lighter assignment; after he left, the assignments were more fair.

The nurse manager eventually had to counsel the staff to stop talking about George so much "because it was interfering with work, not to mention jeopardizing his confidentiality."

In this case, the nurse manager acted responsibly to protect patients' safety, as well as to ensure fair and confidential treatment for George. But doing the right thing also meant that the nurse manager risked the ire of his director and could not rely on her for sound judgment or support. The nurse manager also had to suffer misplaced anger from George and many of the nurses on the unit. "Somebody had to be the target of anger. It couldn't be George, it couldn't be the director, and it couldn't be the doctor. So it was me. It goes with the territory."

It also shows the irony of how the nurses who tried to help George by covering for him and taking care of him, actually put patients at risk of being harmed, and George at risk of being fired for negligence. Although nurses with AIDS need help and understanding, a true friend would have encouraged George to consider the option of going on disability when his dementia was still mild.

John Shared His Diagnosis Early

John likes to work with kids and has continued since he learned in 1984 that he was infected with HIV. He attributes his continuing good health with T-cell counts over 500 to a positive attitude and learning to deal with stress. One way he reduces stress is to be open about his infection at work. "A lot of people now ask me how I'm doing. They seem genuinely happy when my T-cell counts are high. It feels good to know that people care and accept me," he says.

HIV infection has had little direct impact on his nursing. Discussions with his director of nursing and the unit's medical director led to few changes in his practice. Now he wears gloves when he draws bloods, good standard practice for every nurse. "The nursing director also insisted, and I agreed, not to talk about my HIV infection with the patients' families," John adds.

So far, only one family has caused a problem. "I heard second hand that a parent said: 'I don't know what his life is, but he might be gay, he's probably infected with HIV, and I don't want him catheterizing my daughter.' Obviously, I let someone else do it. Families are under enough stress because of their child's illness, and they don't need to have their opinions challenged at that time."

He also informed his nursing director about the incident. She thanked him for the information in case the family decided to talk with her about the matter. She also supported his competence as a nurse and his good judgment in changing the assignment.

John admits that not everyone is supportive, "Some people just back away from me when I talk about HIV. They're horrified." His decision to disclose his HIV infection at work was carefully considered, and he is prepared for any consequence of his disclosure. "I don't like confrontation, but I would fight tooth and nail if I got fired over HIV infection."

LEGAL PROTECTION

Gay and lesbian Americans have more protection from discrimination in employment by being "disabled" with AIDS, than they do as lesbian and gay people. The Americans with Disabilities Act (ADA) outlaws discrimination at work and in places of public accommodation, and the ADA includes HIV infection as a form of disability. The law also requires reasonable modification in the physical plant to accommodate disabled workers (American Civil Liberties Union, undated).

The law hinges on the employee proving he or she can still do the work. For HIV-infected employees, that also means doing the work without putting patients at risk of infection. A judge ruled that a surgical technician could rightfully be transferred to a nonclinical job in the purchasing department because he might infect patients during surgery (Sullivan, 1994).

In another case, a federal court ordered a New York hospital to hire an HIV-infected pharmacist without job restrictions. The hospital had learned of the pharmacist's infection, and as a result, wanted to bar him from mixing IV solutions. An appeals court upheld the ruling. At stake was the hospital's potential loss of $107 million in federal funding if discrimination continued ("Hospital Won't Limit," 1993).

For job applicants, the ADA forbids employers from asking about HIV infection or other medical conditions covered by the ADA, until the employer conditionally offers a job. Although it is permissible to refuse to answer unlawful questions, telling a lie may be suitable grounds for later dismissal. The Gay and Lesbian Medical Association and the National Lawyers Guild advise applicants to avoid voluntarily disclosing their HIV infection unless it is absolutely necessary, but they strongly recommend not to lie (Gautier, 1993).

ANA'S POSITION ON HIV DISEASE

Insiders at the American Nurses Association (ANA) admit with pride that lesbians, gay men, and their heterosexual allies pressed for a humane response to people infected with HIV. "Gay people make sure that AIDS issues are put on the table," says one insider. Thanks to their efforts, the ANA publicly supports access to treatment and research for people infected with HIV, measures to prevent the spread of infection, and nondiscrimination against people with AIDS.

The ANA opposes mandatory HIV-antibody testing and mandatory disclosure. Instead it endorses voluntary confidential testing with informed consent and counseling (ANA, 1993).

After consulting ethicists, the ANA (1993) concluded that nurses infected with HIV are not ethically obligated to disclose their infection to either their employer or their patients, unless a patient is exposed to a reasonable risk of infection. Instead, nurses who know they are infected should avoid performing procedures that put the patient at risk. However, you could be sued for fraud if you tell a patient that you are uninfected when you know that you are infected (Gautier, 1993). The ANA (1993) also recommends that patients be advised of the option of receiving postexposure treatment after a significant exposure. Testing and disclosure are not warranted following trivial exposures.

Even after a patient's exposure, the nurse should remain anonymous from coworkers, insurance carriers, and the patient.

According to the ANA Action Report (1993), "The exposed patient should not be notified of the source's name or exact circumstances of the exposure, but should be given enough information and counseling to fully understand the implications of the event."

HIV infection is not an automatic reason to transfer to a nonclinical assignment. According to an ANA Action Report, "Participation in patient care activities by nursing personnel should not be prohibited solely on the basis of HIV status." Nor is HIV infection sufficient cause to dismiss a student (ANA, 1993).

The ANA (1993) insists that students receive training and protective equipment to keep them safe when caring for patients with blood-borne infections. If students are exposed, schools of nursing should provide postexposure testing, counseling, treatment, and disability coverage for students who prove to be infected. Schools of nursing should also vaccinate students against hepatitis B. To ensure that people with AIDS receive sensitive care, the ANA insists that students learn to give care that "respects client conscience and integrity, cultural values, beliefs, relationships, and the right to make choices."

For nurses exposed to HIV through needle sticks or other work-related injuries, the ANA (1993) provides guidelines for postexposure procedures and how to humanely conduct testing and counseling. As a labor advocate, the ANA encourages state nurses associations to improve worker's compensation insurance for nurses exposed at work.

In 1993, the HIV Task Force of the ANA issued a handbook entitled, *Peer Support for the HIV-Positive Nurse: A Guide for the Development of Programs and Materials* to assist state nurses associations support of HIV-infected members. The ANA (1993) also strongly supports access to health care for all people infected with HIV and calls for an end to discrimination by insurance carriers.

ANAC SUPPORTS NURSES

The Association of Nurses in AIDS Care (ANAC) networks with state and other national nursing organizations to provide support for nurses infected with HIV. At its 1994 national convention,

ANAC held forums for HIV-infected nurses. It continues to evaluate the needs of nurses infected with HIV and develop programs.

NURSES DECRY MANDATORY TESTING

None of the lesbian and gay nurses interviewed support mandatory HIV antibody testing for nurses or any other health care workers. Except when describing individual acts of discrimination, this is the only issue that caused nurses to curse during the interviews.

Gay and lesbian nurses are against mandatory testing first because it does not improve patient care or safety: "I don't agree that it should be mandatory for employment. Universal precautions protect everyone. Most nurses don't put people at risk. I'm more at risk from my patients than they are from me."

Many nurses see mandatory testing as a way to single out and scapegoat nurses: "I'm very much against it. It's wrong for nurses to disclose or be tested when patients don't have to be tested or disclose their antibody status." According to another nurse, "If they will test all patients, then testing nurses is OK. But unless all the physicians and all the patients are tested, then testing nurses is wrong."

Some nurses pointed out the stress of testing: "I'm against mandatory testing for any group. There's no evidence that it slows the spread of the disease, and knowing your status can be damaging when you're not prepared." Another says, "It's not right on a gut level. It could really discriminate."

The opinions of gay and lesbian nurses are in contrast with nurses in general. In a 1992 *RN* survey, 44% of respondents agreed that HIV testing should be mandatory for health care workers. Fully 86% agreed that health care workers who perform exposure-prone procedures should know their HIV and hepatitis B status. However, only 15% of the nurses answered that they would disclose their HIV infection to a patient. More than twice as many, 37%, said they would report a suspected violation, if reporting HIV status were mandatory. However, 91% of the nurses agreed that education and strict adherence to universal precautions are the most effective ways to stop the spread of AIDS (Lippman, 1992a).

ADVICE FOR NURSES INFECTED WITH HIV

Nurses infected with HIV suggest that others who are infected consider the following suggestions:

- ▼ Make disclosure of your HIV infection at work an informed decision. Learn the facts that apply specifically to you, think carefully, then estimate the possible impact of your disclosure on job security and work relationships.
- ▼ Know your employer's benefit package in detail.
- ▼ Change jobs carefully to avoid losing health care and disability because of preexisting conditions.
- ▼ Early in the course of your HIV disease, consider buying supplemental disability insurance.
- ▼ Be positive.
- ▼ Do not reveal your HIV infection unless you are prepared for any possible response. If negative responses would discourage you, then do not disclose.
- ▼ Disclosure is easier if you have already established friendships with coworkers.
- ▼ Everyone infected with HIV responds individually. Expect your mood to fluctuate. Says one nurse, "About the time you think you're OK, you'll get knocked to your knees again."
- ▼ Know your own feelings about being infected before you share your diagnosis with others.
- ▼ Disclose to your friends first and see how you handle their reactions.
- ▼ Before you disclose at work, first gauge your acceptance as a lesbian or gay man.
- ▼ How important is it to be close to the people you work with?
- ▼ Judge the climate. Before you disclose, listen to your coworkers' opinions about AIDS, then decide.
- ▼ If you disclose at work, be prepared for uncomfortable questions.

▾ Be prepared to fight for your job if necessary.

▾ Contact your state nurses association to learn if they provide support services for nurses infected with HIV.

▾ Anonymously contact your state nurses association to determine the reporting requirements for health care professionals who are infected. Regulations differ state by state. Minnesota, for example, requires physicians, health care facilities, and laboratories to report people who are infected with HIV to the state Commissioner of Health. The Commissioner has also recommended that the state legislature change the health professionals practice acts to require HIV-infected licensed professionals to be reported directly to their respective licensing board, and to discipline professionals who fail to report.

▾ For more information and support contact:
The Gay and Lesbian Medical Association
(formerly the American Association of Physicians for Human Rights)
211 Church Street, Suite C
San Francisco, CA 94114
415-864-0408

American Nurses Association
600 Maryland Ave. SW, Suite 100 W
Washington, D.C. 20024-2571
202-554-4444

Association of Nurses in AIDS Care
1555 Connecticut Ave. NW, Suite 200
Washington, D.C. 20036-1103
202-462-1038

CHEMICALLY DEPENDENT NURSES

More nurses lose their licenses because of drug problems—using drugs and alcohol while on duty, stealing drugs at work, or writing illegal prescriptions—than from any other reason. Between 1980 and 1986, the Disciplinary Data Bank of the National Council of State Boards of Nursing reported that 4,319 RNs were disciplined because of drug problems, accounting for 43% of all disciplinary actions. During the same period, 1,811 LPNs were disci-plined because of drug problems, accounting for 34% of all disciplinary action. However, one state reported that 93% of all disciplinary actions against RNs and 95% of actions involving LPNs were related to drug use (Elliot & Heines, 1987).

State Board of Nursing actions represent only the tip of the iceberg. Some nurses use drugs and never get caught, and others wisely seek treatment independently. No one knows exactly how many gay and lesbian nurses are involved. To gain a perspective, compare the incidence of alcohol and drug problems within three overlapping groups—the general population, the gay and lesbian community, and nurses as a whole. Approximately 8 to 10% of the general population abuses alcohol, and 2 to 3% are addicted to drugs (Elliot, 1987).

The rate may be higher but more difficult to estimate for lesbians and gay men. Approximately 30%—three times the rate in the general population—of lesbians and gay men are depen-dent on alcohol or drink excessively, according to the most commonly reported studies (Finnegan & McNally, 1987). Other recent studies estimate 9 to 19% (Singer & Deschamps 1994). Bloomfield (1993), however, reports that randomly selected groups of lesbians and heterosexual women drink similarly. The rate of drug use is not reported, but probably mirrors the rate of alcohol use. Among all nurses, approximately 6 to 16% are impaired due to alcohol or drug use (Lippman, 1992b).

Compared to the general population, more lesbians and gay men need treatment for chemical dependency, and more nurses certainly need treatment. Successful treatment recognizes and nur-tures the nurse's life, including his or her sexual orientation. In order for nurses to provide safe and sober health care, drug rehabilitation programs must be available that are gay and lesbian sensitive.

IMPAIRED PROFESSIONAL PROGRAMS

Until Florida passed the nation's first "diversion" law in 1983, nurses with alcohol and drug problems, regardless of their sexual orientation, were ignored, treated in secrecy, or most often punished—fired, arrested, or denied their license. It is easy to believe that nurses would have been treated more harshly if they were also suspected of being gay or lesbian.

The current emphasis is on treatment or rehabilitation. Each state organizes its own system, administered by the state nurses association, the State Board of Nursing, or an independent agency. Some states have a well-defined program, others only offer referrals, and still others rely on a system of volunteer peer counselors. Lesbian and gay nurses do best where there is a range of options, including services with therapists competent to deal with gay and lesbian issues. The following profiles illustrate the success and limitations of impaired professional programs for lesbian and gay nurses.

PROFILES OF CHEMICALLY DEPENDENT NURSES

The following nurses candidly shared the story of their problems with drugs and alcohol, as well as the hard work and diligence it took to reach and maintain sobriety. Although the nurses were very different—they lived in different parts of the country, selected or were forced into different kinds of treatment, and used different kinds of drugs—they were all heavily influenced by being gay men or lesbians.

Ruth: An Equal Opportunity User

Ruth was caught diverting narcotics at work. She signed out Demerol for a sleeping patient and pocketed the dose. Because it was an ICU, the supervisor was watching the patient sleep, and asked her when the patient woke up to ask for pain medication.

Ruth confessed when her nurse manager called her at home to tell her not to return to work and to ask if she had a drug problem. "She asked if I was alone, and needed help right away. She called me every day. Three days later I met with my manager, supervisor, and an investigator from the State Board of Nursing. I decided I needed help and wrote a confession. They fired me, but agreed to rehire me if I got treatment. I felt relieved that I was going to get help."

She says ICU nurses get caught more because they're more closely observed, not because they use more. "Nurses on general floors use loads of drugs. You can divert for years and not get caught, because it's really easy."

Ruth had a long history of drug and alcohol use. "I switched to narcotics because they were more predictable, easier, and gave me less of a hangover. But I was really an equal opportunity user—alcohol, occasional grass, Valium, and sedatives. I injected whenever it was available: 500 to 600 mg of Demerol per eight-hour shift."

But she did not use drugs every day. "It's more like someone who binge drinks on the weekends. Given the opportunity to use, I would use as much as possible, but not necessarily every day." Doctors, especially the residents, contributed to her problem by writing prescriptions for painkillers and sedatives.

To hide her drug use, she worked the night shift and frequently changed units. "I don't know if there was any suspicion. Only one person commented that I gave a lot of narcotics."

She spent the first 30 days of treatment with inmates, court-mandated people, and others who couldn't afford private treatment. "There was a lesbian counselor who confronted me that I was isolating myself as a lesbian. Part of recovery was realizing that men and other people who were different from me could give me support."

She spent the next nine months in a halfway house. "It could have been a great place. My counselor really understood chemical dependency, but was homophobic. It's very annoying to have to deal with a therapist's homophobia."

For Ruth the issue was not coming out, but dealing with a relationship that was falling apart because of addiction. "If I had been married to a man for eight years, that source of pain in my life would have gotten greater attention. Married women were guided through healing their relationships, or finding a resolution with their loss; where I was ignored."

After the state-mandated program, Ruth found the right therapist. "The most healing thing for me was to find a good therapist who was a lesbian." She also benefited from a 12-step program with other nurses. "The most valuable thing for nurses is to get connected with other nurses who are doing well in 12-step programs. They can uniquely confront the issues and excuses given by other nurses. As time went by, my sponsor, who was gay, talked about how to date and how to have sex sober." Today, she remains active in gay and lesbian AA, and has returned to school to further her career.

Henry Denied His Problem

When Henry regained consciousness in ICU on a ventilator, he still did not believe that he had a drug problem. He was alive only because a neighbor had performed CPR in his apartment two days earlier. The previous week was a blank—lost to alcohol, sedatives, and reefer. "I don't know exactly what I took. I still went to work, and picked up a friend at the airport. But later, my partner told me I went crazy, threw furniture out the window, then had a respiratory arrest."

He started drinking at 17 to numb the pain of an abusive family. "Over the years I tried a lot of drugs to make the pain go away. As a nurse, I learned that I didn't have to drink if I took sedatives. I would steal Valium, Halcion, Dalmane, anything to help me sleep."

A pharmacist enabled his drug abuse. "I took what I wanted and sent the pharmacy a list of what I needed. I never had to falsify records. The pharmacist was gay and sent me extra doses as a favor. One addict helping another."

In ICU, Henry was given the choice of losing his nursing license or entering an impaired professional program. Fortunately, he chose the program: three weeks as an inpatient, five weeks of day hospital, one year of weekly therapy with a psychologist, followed by weekly group meetings, and drug screens for two more years.

But his therapy ignored the possible link between his sexual orientation and his drug use. "I got sober in spite of my treatment. I was told that being gay had nothing to do with chemical dependency, and to leave my gay issues outside of therapy. I got the standard treatment, take it or drink. Standard treatment fails many gay and lesbian nurses." Despite treatment that refused to deal with him as a gay man, Henry has remained sober and drug free.

Helen Drank on Call

When she was on call, Helen started drinking heavily to reduce the isolation and loneliness. She recognized that she had a problem and sought treatment, a seven-week inpatient military program. "The only thing that saved me was the fact that I was a nurse and that meant everything in the world to me, so I got help."

During her intake interview, Helen confided to her counselor that she was a lesbian, and felt that it might influence her treatment. The counselor warned her in no uncertain terms to lie and keep it to herself, or she would suffer for it later. "Even though they were teaching honesty overall, they told me to hide."

Although lying kept her in the military, it was difficult to deal with treatment and hide being a lesbian. "The core of my life had to be left out. I was in a rocky relationship, and I couldn't talk about it in group therapy. I was also drinking to help deal with someone on a sexual level. When you give up drinking, you have to learn how to be a lesbian without drinking. I wasn't able to deal with those issues until much later." Helen, like many addicted lesbian and gay nurses, was left on her own to find what may have been the most significant part of her treatment. She remains sober, is in a committed relationship, and continues to practice as a nurse practitioner.

Tod Started Using Socially

Methamphetamine injected intravenously was Tod's drug of choice. "It allowed me to have a personality I wouldn't otherwise have— talkative and outgoing—where I'm really a shy, country boy." He started using in his early twenties, casually at first at small parties. Within a year, he was injecting daily, and eventually he could not work. "Instead of going to work, I wanted to stay home and get high. Only at the very end did I use at work." Tod turned himself in and was treated through a peer-assistance program.

Although he is comfortable with being gay, he admits that being gay helped him to use. "It was important to stay up all night, to be social, popular, accepted. And crystal is freely available in the gay community. Being a nurse also helped. I had free access to needles, and I developed excellent technique at giving IV injections. Being a nurse also prevented me from seeking treatment sooner—I thought a nurse couldn't be an addict."

Fortunately, he was directed to a program with other nurses. "The gay thing kept coming up, but it was OK to talk about gay things, even though I was the only gay man in the group."

Later Tod became very involved in the lesbian and gay AA network. "In the first part of my treatment, it was more important to be with other nurses, later it was more important to be with other gay people." During recovery, Tod fell in love with a new lover; and they have built a life together for the past seven years. He went back to school in nursing administration and now is a sober, drug-free nurse manager.

Valerie Diverted Narcotics

Valerie also got caught diverting narcotics at work. She started drinking when she was 16 years old. By 18 she was drinking daily and would binge when she could get away with it. Soon after, she started smoking pot every day. "I was in a relationship with an alcoholic, and I hid behind her. No matter how much I drank, she drank more, so I looked good."

Things got worse after she had major surgery and had a PCA unit for pain. "Demerol became my best friend." Then she started diverting by skimming the remainder of Demerol doses for patients. She started by giving herself IM injections, but soon that was not enough:

> IVs were my specialty, so I started injecting intravenously. At first, I did it by the book, diluted it in the right amount of solution, and injected slow IV push over three to five minutes. But eventually I just gave it as quickly as I could, and mixed Demerol with morphine and leftover Benedryl, Phenergan, or Vistaril. I was injecting one to five times a day, 400 to 500 mg of Demerol total. Most of the nurses I know in treatment are Demerol addicts.

A coworker got suspicious when a patient Valerie supposedly medicated did not get the expected pain relief. Her director called her into her office. "I had one pocket full of clean syringes and the other filled with Demerol. I stuffed the syringes in the trash and the Demerol in the sharps container." She was confronted with a record of the narcotics she had dispensed and decided to come clean. She was terminated and entered into a diversion program.

Valerie and her intake counselor together decided on an appropriate therapy placement. If random urine drug screens are positive, the nurse is switched to another program, or admitted to an inpatient unit. "You pick the program, and they'll accept it as long as it's a real program. Because my supervisor was a lesbian, she was guiding me in ways that suited me as a lesbian without me even knowing it."

She went on disability and entered a sober-living home. For nine months, she had therapy sessions five times daily, then decreased to three times weekly. Thirteen months later she returned to work with stipulations aimed at keeping her drug-free—no night shifts, no giving narcotics, limited patient care, and no responsibility for the narcotics keys. In total, the program lasted from two to five years with random urine tests 18 times a year.

She explains how lesbian and gay bars contributed to her problem. "When I came out, I was already drinking. But after coming out, it's easy to stay in your problem. Where do you go to hang out? A bar. Where do you meet people? A bar. Where can you go to be yourself? A bar. Coming out was easy, but bars made it easy to stay in the problem. It's sad."

Valerie got help from an outpatient group limited to women. Some of the patients and counselors were out lesbians. "If a greater number of my issues were lesbian issues, I don't think it would have been nearly enough. I would still be dog paddling around."

Unlike the other nurses interviewed, Valerie does not recommend AA. "I can't stand gay and lesbian AA meetings. I see a lot of gays and lesbians go to AA and stay sober for a couple of months, then get drunk."

For Valerie, her lesbian-related issues were a small part of her recovery. "There are so many things that are more important than our sexuality. We all have a past, including emotional abuse. Our sexuality issues fall into place after we deal with the other issues, such as incest. I don't believe that gays and lesbians are terminally unique. We don't have more significant needs than the general population."

However, she needed help dealing with her relationship. "I was in a really bad relationship with a woman, and I realized that there was no one to talk to about our relationship. Gay and lesbian relationships have unique characteristics. I felt isolated. Although the counselor was a lesbian, she wasn't much help."

Valerie also echoed the importance of finding treatment with other nurses. "If you're the only nurse, you're separate. Other addicts don't see you as the same as them. For one thing, you do prescription drugs, and that's different."

She also stresses the importance of honesty. "If you're honest with people about being a lesbian, you'll get better treatment." Today she is working her way back into nursing practice. Her program still dictates the kind of unit she can work on, and limits her to the day shift. But most importantly, her random drug tests remain negative.

SELECTING SENSITIVE TREATMENT

The Pride Institute, a leader in alcohol and drug treatment for lesbians, gay men, and bisexuals, developed the following set of questions to ask when considering a treatment center:

1. Is your facility accredited by the Joint Commission on Accreditation of Healthcare Organizations?

2. Is this a lesbian and gay treatment center or just a "gay track" or sideline program at a "straight" hospital? Do you operate a "Christian Program" in your facility?

3. What do you mean by "gay and lesbian program"? Will I be housed with lesbian or gay people and be in all

gay or lesbian groups, or will all the groups be mixed together depending on the number of patients in the "gay and lesbian program"? If in mixed groups, how can the group members' prejudices be handled? Will I be able to speak about the most important parts of my life?

4. How many lesbian and gay patients are in your facility today?

5. Is this a psychiatric hospital or a drug and alcohol treatment center? Will I be locked up?

6. How long has this "gay or lesbian program" been in business? What is your success rate? Ask to see an independent outcome study.

7. How much will this hospital charge my insurance company? Will I have any benefits for continuing therapy after I am discharged?

8. Will my counselor be lesbian or gay? What is her/his education background, years of experience?

9. Has this hospital, or its parent company, been charged with or investigated for any fraudulent or deceptive practices?

(Copyright © 1993 Pride Institute. Reprinted with permission.)

TREATMENT ISSUES

Lesbians and gay men may not be "terminally unique," as one nurse put it, but at some point in treatment, gay or lesbian issues require attention.

  ▾ A low sense of self-worth: many gay men and lesbians have been told repeatedly by church, family, school, and society that they have little worth and need to change. Society victimizes lesbians and gay men.

  ▾ A high rate of physical, emotional, and sexual abuse, including incest among both men and women. A study at the Pride Institute found that nearly 50% of gay men and lesbians receiving treatment at the Institute reported past sexual abuse (Neisen & Sandall, 1990). Their treatment for chemical dependency required exploration of their sexual abuse issues.

▼ Because of loneliness, lesbians and gay men may enter dysfunctional relationships. During treatment, they need help dealing with relationship issues, especially relationships that are ending.

▼ Some gay men and lesbians can only confront their sexual needs when they are intoxicated, and they may never have had sex sober. Learning to meet people and have sex sober is a major treatment goal.

▼ HIV infection may complicate treatment. Some people use alcohol and drugs to deal with the pain and fear of AIDS.

▼ Coming out issues frequently surface during treatment. Some people use alcohol and drugs to avoid confronting their sexual orientation; and until they are sober, they may be unable to determine their sexual orientation. Some people must be intoxicated to maintain an ostensibly heterosexual lifestyle. Closeted people need help coming out.

▼ Alcohol and drug use is influenced by all the issues of life, including relationships, discrimination, and conflict over sexual orientation.

▼ Most people abuse a combination of drugs and alcohol.

▼ Finding alternatives to bars as places to meet people may be difficult in some gay and lesbian communities.

▼ AA may be unacceptable to some people for a variety of reasons.

▼ Discrimination based on sexual orientation can sabotage treatment.

▼ Many delay seeking treatment because they fear discrimination.

- ▼ Therapists must be fluent in gay and lesbian cultures, as well as being skilled as chemical dependency counselors.

- ▼ Lesbians and gay men are entitled to group therapy where they can fully participate without prejudice.

ADVICE FOR CHEMICALLY DEPENDENT NURSES

Nurses in recovery from drug and alcohol problems give the same advice: admit that you have a problem and find help. The following suggestions might make it easier:

- ▼ Get help as soon as possible. You probably have more options by voluntarily seeking treatment.

- ▼ Find a sensitive treatment program by networking through the gay and lesbian communities. Contact your community center or hotline and talk with people in recovery. The Gay Yellow Pages lists therapists by state and city. Your local lesbian or gay newspaper may also list local services. The Pride Institute, 612-934-7554, can also suggest local resources.

- ▼ Visit a program and ask: How do you deal with gay men or lesbians? Do you treat other nurses? How many nurses are in the program?

- ▼ Avoid programs where you have to hide your sexual orientation.

- ▼ Contact your state nurses association or State Board of Nursing to find rehabilitation programs.

- ▼ Contact your employer's benefits department to access employee assistance programs and to determine if voluntary treatment is covered by your medical or disability insurance.

- ▼ If you are subject to criminal charges or disciplinary action by your State Board of Nursing, you are entitled to due process and legal counsel. In many states, but not all states, disciplinary action must be related to the practice of nursing, rather than criminal charges such as driving under the influence of alcohol or possession of narcotics during nonworking hours.

▾ Recovering sober nurses are protected from discrimination in hiring by the Americans with Disabilities Act (ADA). However, the ADA does not protect nurses currently abusing drugs or alcohol.

SUMMARY

HIV infects more nurses because of personal sexual and drug habits than because of occupational exposures. Unfortunately, gay men are disproportionately affected and require support and legal protection from discrimination. Lesbian and gay nurses have led the profession in providing humane care for people with AIDS.

Compared to HIV infection, more nurses struggle with chemical dependency or alcohol problems. Because of the stress, availability of drugs, and isolation of working long and unpredictable hours, nurses are at risk. Gay men and lesbians are at greater risk. Too frequently, treatment programs tacitly assume that everyone in treatment is heterosexual, which sabotages gay men and lesbians from seeking or benefiting from treatment. Lesbian and gay nurses deserve the same treatment that heterosexual nurses take for granted—treatment that recognizes who they are, the relationships they value, and the communities they live in.

References

American Civil Liberties Union. (undated). *The Americans with disabilities act: What it means for people living with HIV disease, questions and answers.* New York: Author.

American Nurses Association. (1993). *Compendium of HIV/AIDS position statements, policies, and documents.* Washington, DC: American Nurses Publishing.

Bloomfield, K. (1993). A comparison of alcohol consumption between lesbians and heterosexual women in an urban population. *Drug and Alcohol Dependence, 33*(3), 257–269.

Centers for Disease Control and Prevention. (1995). First 500,000 AIDS cases — United States, 1995. *Morbidity and Mortality Weekly Report, 44*(46), 849–853.

Eliason, M., Donelan, C., & Randall, C. (1992). Lesbian stereotypes. *Health Care for Women International, 13*(2), 131–144.

Elliot, R. L., & Heines, M. J. (1987). *Disciplinary data bank: A longitudinal study.* Chicago: National Council of State Boards of Nursing, Inc.

Finnegan, D. G., & McNally, E. B. (1987). *Dual identities: Counseling chemically dependent gay men and lesbians.* Center City, MN: Hazelden.

Gautier, E. (1993). *The legal rights and obligations of HIV-infected health care workers.* San Francisco: American Association of Physicians for Human Rights and New York: the National Lawyers Guild.

Hospital Won't Limit Duties of HIV+ Pharmacist. (1993). *RN, 55*(4), 18–19.

Latest CDC Stats Hint at Nurses' Vulnerability to HIV. (1994). *RN, 57*(4), 17.

Lippman, H. (1992a). HIV and professional ethics: Nurses speak out. *RN, 55*(6), 28–32.

Lippman, H. (1992b). Addicted nurses: Tolerated, tormented, or treated? *RN, 55*(4), 36–41.

Neisen, J. H., & Sandall, H. (1990). Alcohol and other drug abuse in a gay/lesbian population: Related to victimization? *Journal of Psychology & Human Sexuality, 3*(1), 151–168.

Raiteri, R., Fora, R., & Sinicco, A. (1994). No HIV-1 transmission through lesbian sex. *The Lancet, 344*(8917), 270.

Singer, B. L., & Deschamps, D. (Eds.). (1994). *Gay and lesbian stats: A pocket guide of facts and figures.* New York: The New Press.

Sullivan, G. H. (1994). Your rights when you're disabled—and afterward. *RN, 57*(8), 61–63.

7 NURSING STUDENTS

Nursing holds up this checklist of what makes a good nurse, and many of the things that I am are not on the list. So I have to seek a lot of outside support that I will be a good nurse. I'm going to be a good nurse because I'm a lesbian, not in spite of the fact that I'm a lesbian.

A lesbian student

Try not to separate your life into compartments that can't be integrated. Yet remain sensitive to the culture around you. Seek out mentors from the camaraderie of a minority group. Don't pick someone just because they're gay, but because they can understand the complexity of your life.

A national nursing leader and lesbian

RESPONSIBILITIES TO STUDENTS

All colleges should be expected to offer students: (1) a comprehensive professional body of knowledge, (2) positive role models, (3) resources for students to maintain health and well-being, (4) freedom from harm, and (5) an environment that encourages intellectual curiosity and emotional growth. For lesbian and gay nursing students, most schools abdicate their responsibilities.

COMING OUT

Coming out in nursing school may be more difficult than coming out at work or to family members. Margaret went to nursing school right out of high school. She chose a large state university with a good reputation, yet her classmates and instructors were unsupportive when she came out. "The students were horrified. When I came out, I confided in an instructor that I trusted. I told her because coming out was pretty frightening. She told me to go to church. I felt abandoned. She didn't refer me to the gay and lesbian advocacy group."

A gay man had a similar experience. He says, "It's important to find a support person on faculty, but I picked the wrong one. She told me I should seek a counselor to help me become straight." Another adult learner says, "It's really lonely and alienating because I can't identify a single ally."

Reasons for Coming Out

A few students cited activist reasons for coming out at school. "If you feel safe, come out. You can be a teacher and prevent homophobia. Talk about it in class discussions, and other people can learn from you." Another student stresses coming out to friends for the same reason. "If it's possible, be out and allow your fellow students to explore a different culture through friendship with you."

A 20-year-old lesbian says, "It's difficult not to be out in nursing school. I feel guilty. But the intellectual side says you have a responsibility to yourself, and you do what it takes to get through. What's more important, getting through this program, or changing this program? It's unfair that I should have to worry about this."

Deciding Not to Come Out

Almost every nursing student describes nursing school as a hostile and dangerous environment for lesbians and gay men. Even students who are otherwise out feel that they must hide in their nursing program. "I'm out in every other aspect of my life, but I feel so insecure at school. I usually feel very comfortable with being out. Everybody already thinks I am weird, and I don't want to be viewed as weirder."

One student is emphatic about not coming out: "Keep your mouth shut until you get a job and become established. You're more vulnerable because of grades." Another agrees, "Coming out could endanger my staying in school. They always call it something else. Inside I hate staying in the closet. It's like turning your back on your own." An adult student advises, "Students have to test the waters more gingerly. Nursing school is not a good place for 18-year-olds to come out."

Even students who are somewhat older and more mature in their lesbian or gay identity agonize about whether to come out at school. A gay man who entered nursing school in his late 30s says, "It's stressful enough being a nursing student—long hours, little sleep—and you add the stress of coming out, and I think it's very hard." One lesbian student says:

> I don't want to be somebody's reference point or role model. It's a burden. I just want to be seen as a human being. If there were another lesbian, I'd be more out. I kind of feel like a traitor. I ask myself if I'm ashamed of myself. I enjoy the closeness that's so easy, so nice, so supportive when women don't worry about you being a lesbian. It's happened before. When I come out, it changes the relationship. You can feel the withdrawal.

Some students do not come out because their classmates are narrow-minded and inexperienced. A returning adult student who chose not to come out says, "When you come out, you have the responsibility to answer their questions and be available to them. I don't have the energy to do that all the time, but that's my only reason for not coming out." Another student recalls, "I didn't want to reveal to them. The main focus of their lives was boyfriends and marriages, but I was afraid to tell the truth."

Applying as an Out Student

The first decision about coming out occurs during the admission process. A lesbian who sits on the admissions board of her college is emphatic, "If it was close between you and someone else, then you'd lose. The level of education doesn't matter. If you're an undergraduate, graduate, or PhD student, don't come out before you're admitted."

An experienced academic says, "If I really needed to get in that program, I would not come out openly, unless I got some clues that it was OK." Another warns, "Don't do anything to jeopardize your placement in a program."

A student recently accepted to a doctoral program did not follow the advice to remain closeted. "My job—seven years in a gay and lesbian health clinic—comes out for me. If that isn't enough, then I refer to my partner. Or I explain my interest in AIDS—as a lesbian, it affects my community. I feel more natural and easier. It's who I am, take it or leave it."

Empowerment

Several students described the strength that comes from knowing who they are as a lesbian or gay person, regardless of their decision to come out. "You didn't choose it," explains a student. "In the end, be true to yourself. Being gay has nothing to do with your performance as a nurse, except that you know what it feels like to be a minority. I think it makes us better."

A young gay man says, "Be honest with yourself. Read a lot about homosexuality, and be in touch with your feelings." A returning lesbian student agrees, "You have to be comfortable with who you are, then you can be out at nursing school. Most straight kids are oblivious, and being out educates them."

An LPN student put it this way, "Be your own best friend. If you're in a small town, you have to rely on yourself. If you're happy with yourself, don't let anyone change who you are."

A lesbian educator focuses on students' self-esteem rather than if they are out. She explains, "Learn as much as you can from each clinical situation. If you're hassled for being gay, then this too shall pass, and next semester you'll have a new instructor. If you don't feel that your love and your worth as a person are as good as everyone else's, then I'll remind students. It might make a difference to hear it from a faculty person."

STUDENT ATTITUDES

Almost all the students complained of narrow-minded attitudes expressed by their classmates. "They couldn't take care of AIDS patients because of their lifestyle, or attend a birth when the mother was lesbian, or care for someone getting an abortion because of religious indignation."

Another says, "My classmates are at ground zero in terms of gay issues. They don't understand treating partners as part of the family and including partners in care. They also don't know all the silent minorities whose values they're offending."

A lesbian student expected more from her classmates. She says, "In a helping profession, I expected more people to understand all walks of life, and deal with issues of sexuality. I was disappointed that nursing students aren't accepting. I would like to see students want to learn more about us."

An instructor from the Midwest agrees, "Some of my students would respond that they couldn't care for a gay patient because it's a sin. I'd show a video depicting gay and lesbian patients, and I would have to stop the video because of giggling and insulting remarks."

A student describes bigoted comments made in a class discussion. She reports that her classmates said, "Gay people aren't normal, and it's ridiculous that gay people are fighting for their rights. It's not part of God's plan."

A lesbian student attributes her classmates' bigoted attitudes in part to the rigor of nursing school. She says, "The environment is very cliquey and very competitive. After high school, they get right into nursing, and it's a hard program, and they don't have time to explore other areas."

However, a gay man who went to a small college right out of high school and came out as a freshman had a different experience. The college is known for its liberal environment, and the general student attitudes helped him. He says, "It was laid back, anything goes, you were free to experience the full range. I developed a strong support system of students—gay, lesbian, and cool straight people."

Researchers (Eliason, Donelan, & Randall, 1992) surveyed nursing students about lesbian stereotypes. The students felt that lesbians were too blatant, wanted to be men, seduced nonlesbian women, were a bad influence on children, and spread disease. In another study, 50% of nursing students said that a lesbian lifestyle was not acceptable, 15% thought that lesbian sex should be illegal, and only 24% would invite a lesbian into their home (Eliason & Randall, 1991). Sadly, nursing students are no better informed or accepting of diversity than the general public, and nursing school does little to change their opinions.

FACULTY ATTITUDES

A lesbian nursing student sized up her instructors, "I felt that a handful of nursing instructors had this military vibe, and I got this real sick homophobia feeling. These nurses had this air of power and homophobia. They were women in power who had no respect for women. My instructors were nurses who didn't really know how to teach."

A lesbian instructor describes the stereotypic remarks made by her peers during a faculty meeting:

> An instructor who identifies herself as a born-again says that she is concerned that one of the male nurses in the clinical unit was making passes at a male student. "You know he's that way. How can I protect him?" Without realizing it, she outed the staff nurse, and repeated a stereotype of molestation. Another instructor said, "I know how to solve the gay problem. Enlist all gay people and put them on the front lines." In other words: Kill us.

Many instructors still believe that men in nursing must be gay. A lesbian instructor says, "If the man is married, then they feel comfortable, and it's OK. But if the man is gay, they feel challenged sometimes to the core of their values."

A lesbian faculty member notes, "If you're doing something weird, like being gay, then 75% of the faculty will gossip about it. Nursing faculty by and large are opinionated, negative, judgmental bigots. I think that they believe that by being professionals they have an ability to make these judgments."

Many students are disappointed that their instructors do not act professionally. An instructor says, "PhDs are no different than anyone else, except that in general they are more narrow-minded than anyone else."

Many of these comments confirm survey results from BSN educators in the Midwest (Randall, 1989). Their responses indicate that 24% of instructors think that lesbian behavior is wrong, 23% think it is immoral, 15% think it is perverted, 34% think it is disgusting, and 19% think it should remain illegal. Instructors maintain stereotypic and inaccurate beliefs: 20% believe that lesbians are a common source of transmitting AIDS, 9% think that lesbianism itself is a disease that can be cured, and 17% think that lesbians molest children. Surprisingly, 28% think they would have difficulty talking with a known lesbian, and 14% would object if their child or a friend's child were being cared for by a lesbian nurse. It is little wonder that lesbian students are reluctant to disclose their sexual orientation and frequently feel like outsiders.

A student points out the most important aspect of faculty attitudes. "Attitudes of faculty trickle down to students, then trickle down to attitudes toward gay and lesbian patients, who don't access care because they feel the nurse's negative attitudes. A big red light goes on, you have to deal with attitudes."

Allies on Faculty

A few students described nonlesbian or gay instructors who supported them. Paul came out to his instructor following a troublesome incident: "A patient's wife was cold towards me and judgmental about AIDS. She fished around to ask if I had a girlfriend. I responded that nurses care for people without judging them. Then I asked my instructor for a break to cool off." He explained the situation to his instructor who responded unexpectedly. She said, "I just want you to know that God loves you. You did a good job, and you'll make a good nurse."

SUPPORTING STUDENTS

Supporting gay and lesbian nursing students can be complicated because of the wide variety of life experiences that gay and lesbian students bring to school. There are at least four very distinct groups: (1) adolescents who came out, at least to themselves, in high school, and are fairly confident, (2) adolescents who are exploring their sexual orientation and come out while in nursing school, (3) mature students who are exploring their sexual orientation in nursing school, and (4) mature students who are secure in the ways they express their sexual orientation.

Instructors can offer appropriate support by understanding the stages of coming out. The six-stage model proposed by Cass (1979) is one theoretic schema of coming out. These broad guidelines need to be tailored to fit a student's unique experience.

Stage 1: Identity Confusion

Students in this stage need positive role models and prejudice-free classroom and clinical environments. Use patient examples from a broad range of cultural groups, but avoid cultural stereotypes. Monitor and provide a counterpoint to student comments that express prejudice. Avoid any comment that gives the impression that instructors gossip about students.

Stage 2: Identity Comparison

Besides role models and an environment free of prejudice, students in this stage need an understanding distance. They may be moody or confused and feel uncomfortable discussing sexual issues. If you suspect a student is lesbian or gay, avoid outing him or her by making undue eye contact while discussing gay or lesbian issues, or by asking their opinion. Out faculty may seem intimidating or inspiring to people in this stage. It may be too soon to suggest attending support groups. Students may feel very threatened by gossiping and pejorative joking, because they feel that they are being secretly judged. Students may benefit from lesbian-and-gay-sensitive counseling, but they seek help because they feel confused and cannot yet identify a need to deal with their sexual orientation.

Stage 3: Identity Tolerance

Students in this stage need certainty and ample feedback that they are OK. It is unlikely that they will come out to an instructor; but if they do, it should be treated delicately. These students are vulnerable and want reassurance. They want to be treated like everyone else. Even when it becomes obvious that students are lesbian or gay, avoid outing them by asking their opinion in class. Students in this stage may be very sensitive to bigoted remarks by students and faculty. Turmoil over coming out may interfere with academic performance. Students may also benefit from confidential counseling or support groups.

Stage 4: Identity Acceptance

At this stage, students need to talk about their new life, loves, and insights. They may volunteer to take the gay or lesbian point of view in class discussions. While it is important to acknowledge their new identity, it is equally important to honor their need to determine the level of intimacy at school. They may still want to separate their personal life from their school life. As they explore their new community, their academic performance may slip because they do not have enough time to meet the conflicting time demands of school and friends.

Stage 5: Identity Pride

During this stage, some students act the most stereotypically. They thrive in lesbian and gay student groups. They are almost compelled to bring up gay and lesbian issues in class, and they will confront bigotry. They also want to improve the treatment of gay men and lesbians by ensuring that their issues are raised in class whenever possible. Other students may feel that lesbian and gay students are monopolizing the discussion. Instructors can avoid this conflict by publicly acknowledging the issue, including diverse patient examples, and encouraging diverse points of view. Trying to suppress gay and lesbian issues during class discussions only makes students in this stage more vocal. Students may insist on wearing obvious symbols of lesbian or gay identity. If possible, offer students in this stage clinical experiences with gay or lesbian patients. During earlier stages, asking the student to write a paper on AIDS or lesbian parents would have felt too threatening; now gay or lesbian topics are welcomed. Students need to know that the rules of conduct are the same for all students regardless of sexual orientation.

Stage 6: Identity Synthesis

Students in this stage may be very quiet about their sexual orientation. They are not afraid of being identified as gay or lesbian, but they recognize that nursing school may be a hostile environment that does not honor intimate information about students. They may confront obviously prejudicial statements in class discussions, and they will not tolerate bigotry. A few may choose to be informal teachers for others about lesbian and gay issues, but many view nursing school as a temporary job that does not require coming out. They are also very skilled at assessing the social landscape to know how to succeed as a lesbian or gay person.

FACULTY STRATEGIES

Theresa Stephany (1992) suggested a continuum of strategies for lesbian and gay faculty, as well as their allies, to take to improve gay and lesbian sensitivity and promote diversity on campus. These strategies range from low-risk to high-risk actions.

Low Risk

▾ Investigate your school's statement of nondiscrimination. Does it include sexual orientation? If not, get it changed.

▾ Show and discuss the commercially available video *Torch Song Trilogy* when teaching family theory.

▾ Discuss alternative lifestyles in required nursing courses.

▾ Gay and lesbian youth are at high risk for suicide. Include this information in your psychiatric/mental health course and incorporate it when counseling students.

Moderate Risk

▾ Discuss homophobia at a faculty meeting.

▾ Campaign and vote for legislators who support anti-discriminatory legislation and encourage others to do the same.

▾ Form a support group for gay/lesbian students within the nursing department.

▾ Meet other supporters of lesbian and gay rights by attending a local meeting of Parents and Friends of Lesbians and Gays (PFLAG). Consult the phone directory to locate chapters.

▾ Encourage students to query prospective employers about their nondiscriminatory policies and then select employers who guarantee equal protection to all minority nurses.

High Risk

▾ Mandate your department curriculum committee to ensure that all course content reflects varied lifestyles and sexual orientations.

▾ Be political. March in the next Gay/Lesbian Freedom Day Parade held across the nation.

▾ Refuse to allow recruiters from all branches of the military access to nursing students until the military reverses its policy of discrimination based solely on sexual orientation.

▾ Introduce a resolution to the college/university's academic senate calling for removal of campus-based ROTC programs that actively discriminate against gay/lesbian students.

▾ Demand domestic partners contract language in your professional contract.

▾ If you are a gay/lesbian faculty member, consider coming out to your students and peers.

(Reprinted with permission.)

SUPPORT DURING CLINICALS

Clinical practice can raise issues that students struggle to put into a professional perspective. They may be exposed to very intimate events, horrible sights, personal tragedies, and abusive or inappropriate patients. Nongay students rely on their instructors for support and guidance. Lesbian and gay students do not always feel the same sense of safety to seek support.

Helen remembers an incident that occurred while she was learning how to do pelvic exams. "A disfigured woman started cooing during the pelvic exam. I was mortified. I was practically in tears. I questioned if I had crossed boundaries. I assumed it was because I was gay, not because of the patient's issues. I questioned if I wanted to be a nurse."

Instead of relying on her instructor for help, Helen was isolated by fear:

> I didn't share this with the instructor because she already wanted to get me and would have used it as an opportunity to kick me out. Instead, I used my personal network and talked with friends. They helped me think it through from the patient's point of view. I realized that it had more to do with the patient's needs, than with me being a lesbian. Now I put a big wall up that prevents me from seeing patients as sexual. It's my wall, and I need it. I'm still caring, but professional.

Another student, who had been out longer, intentionally kept sexual issues hidden from his instructors because "it was already taken care of, and they would have had a heart attack, they wouldn't have been able to deal with it." He explains, "A patient put his hand on my knee and asked for my phone number so that we could get together. I said that wouldn't be professional, that I've come too far, and have too much to lose. I gave him the number of the gay hotline and the MCC."

DISCRIMINATION AGAINST STUDENTS

Most nursing students sense the potential hostility in nursing schools and do not come out because they fear discrimination. A gay educator says, "At smaller, more mediocre, ordinary schools, there is homophobia and discrimination against gays. Most of the colleges in our area are closety and backwards."

Frequently, students and faculty report that the university is more supportive than the college of nursing. A nursing professor explains, "At my school, the university as a whole is better at supporting gay and lesbian students than is the college of nursing. We have an excellent counseling program. All of the counselors are safe zones."

Safe zones guarantee that the designated space will be free of harassment. Members of the gay and lesbian community or campus organization conduct workshops for instructors and put a decal on the door, indicating that it is a safe place for lesbians and gay men. In some colleges, faculty and students wear buttons indicating that they uphold the principles of maintaining a safe zone.

Grading is not standardized, at least in the view of students. A recent graduate from a nursing school in the South advises students to think twice before coming out because they might be punished for it. She remembers, "A man was called into the director's office and told to keep his sexuality to himself. And he did. Clinicals are graded totally subjectively, and if they wanted to fail someone, it would be easy."

One student hired a lawyer to fight the school's decision that he would have to repeat a year because he failed a psychology class. In his eyes, the reasons were trumped up and based on bigotry. Although the conflict was resolved by repeating the class during the summer, the experience exacted a personal toll. "When I failed, I went through a deep depression. I thought I might commit suicide. I couldn't believe that it was happening because I was gay. I was such a good student. I always got *A*s in class and clinics. I didn't know who I could trust after that."

A woman describes her experience with a bigoted and abusive instructor, "Another student and I, we were both lesbians, had to do a makeup clinical. The instructor screamed for the first hour about how we weren't nurse material. Luckily, we weren't 18-year-olds, and we could tolerate this abuse. We finished school."

A gay man who first attended a diploma school left during his last term because of discrimination. "Six months before graduation, I was told that I wasn't RN material. We were treated like children. All three gay men failed OB together. They failed us in the clinical." He enrolled in a university and graduated without a problem. He concludes that being gay was the only reason he was not RN material at the first school.

Hate Speech and Violence

Verbal and physical abuse are common experiences for gay and lesbian university students. In a study at Yale University (Herek, 1993), as a result of being lesbian or gay, 65% of the respondents had been the targets of insults, 25% had been threatened with violence; and 42% had been the victims of physical abuse, such as being chased, having things thrown at them, or having their property damaged.

A survey in Illinois (Duncan, 1990) showed that the prevalence of sexual assault for university students is higher among women than among men. But it is also higher for lesbians and gay men than for heterosexuals.

A 20-year-old lesbian nursing student says, "It's hard when you realize that your fellow students are so insensitive. They use hate words. They say, 'That's so queer, that's so gay.' It means that's dumb or stupid."

DISCRIMINATION AGAINST FACULTY

Lesbian and gay faculty, as well as students, can be the victims of discrimination. An instructor who was not offered an opportunity to renew her contract explains, "One of the reasons I lost my last teaching job was that my boss was no longer interested in supporting me as a lesbian. I was forbidden to bring up gay or lesbian issues in small group discussions, unless the client brought it up directly to the student, which would never happen. I was furious. The students complained that these discussions were upsetting."

Another instructor says, "There are ways to make it so that you can't proceed. You're glad if people would just say it out loud. I wasn't getting teaching jobs that I was well qualified for. Suddenly they didn't have openings. It felt annihilating. It eats away at your inner self-esteem and confidence."

CULTURAL COMPETENCE

Nursing as a profession insists that patients receive culturally competent care, but few nursing schools give students the tools to practice it. A doctoral candidate says, "There's a lot of lip service paid, but it's just lip service, because of the people assigned to teach it."

An instructor in another university agrees, "Cultural diversity is supposed to be one of the themes running through the entire curriculum, but there's no mention of gay issues, just ethnic content. The class on sexuality focuses only on heterosexualism."

A West Coast instructor says, "Lip service isn't enough. It means getting in there and struggling with those issues. You don't get it from a one-hour lecture on cultural diversity. You don't get it from reading a book. Nursing needs more hands-on experience of acceptance. Identify what you value, and how you express that in your practice."

Students also question the quality of the instruction they receive concerning cultural diversity. "They talk about a multicultural perspective, but I haven't met a teacher yet who can tell me what that really means," says a student at a prestigious university. "They have a poor grasp on making it real for anyone."

The solution, according to an experienced professor, is faculty development. "The nursing faculty is a little smug. They think they already do it. But when it comes to application, there's a lot missing. Faculty need to be desensitized. It's a lot of work to get students to go beyond the obvious. In nursing, we have to bring diversity into every course through case studies."

She also advocates examining student attitudes: "We need to develop strategies to address very conservative students to become more tolerant. Now that conservatives are in Congress, closeted conservative students are being more vocal. We should discuss the ethics of nurses who do not follow the code of ethics because of narrow-mindedness. I'm trying to learn to bring people's attitudes out early."

Milton Bennett (1986) described six stages of intercultural sensitivity from denial to integration. In terms of lesbian and gay cultures, many nursing instructors are still in the first stage, denial. They isolate themselves to preclude contact with cultural differences, they describe gay men and lesbians in terms of broad categories, or they attribute the cultural differences to a sub-human or perverted status. Some are in the second, or defense, stage. They espouse negative stereotypes and assume that gay and lesbian cultures are inferior. Few, if any, reach the highest stage called integration. In this stage, instructors are able to shift cultural world views to put themselves in the place of a lesbian or gay man and evaluate the ethics of a situation from that person's point of view. According to Bennett, people in this stage of development "experience differences as an essential and joyful aspect of life."

A student explains the connection between cultural diversity and the absence of openly lesbian or gay role models on faculty. "There's a lot of lip service paid to a liberal philosophy of acceptance. When the subject of gay and lesbians comes up, like with families, they include it; but there's no out lesbian on the faculty. The message is rampantly heterosexual. It's inexcusable that there's no out gay or lesbian faculty to act as a role model and a resource for other faculty."

In many nursing colleges, the solution to the cultural diversity problem involves a class devoted to the topic. One student, who served in the Peace Corps and received sophisticated cross-cultural training, criticizes his nursing class. "It was limited to a cookbook formula, yet another list of things to memorize: Asian-Americans do this, and African-Americans do that. It was offensive, and sent many people around the bend. I would have preferred having members of the cultural group represent the group."

Some students regretted that because of the risk of coming out, they could not act as resources for their classmates about lesbian and gay issues. One student says, "If we could be out at school, I could talk about being gay. There's a whole new light that I could help people see, if they were willing to look."

American Academy of Nursing Recommendations

In 1992, an expert panel of the American Academy of Nursing (AAN) recognized gay men and lesbians among the groups requiring culturally competent care. The panel also recommended the following principles to prepare nursing students to deliver competent care to any minority group:

▾ A nurse must learn to appreciate intergroup and intragroup cultural differences and commonalities in racial/ethnic minority populations.

▾ A nurse must understand how social structural factors shape health behaviors and practices in racial/ethnic minorities; for example, it is important for nurses to avoid a "blaming and victim" ideology.

▾ A nurse must understand the dynamics and challenges in biculturalism and bilingualism where groups may live and function in two cultures.

▾ Nurses must confront their own ethnocentrism and racism.

▾ Nurses must begin rehearsing, practicing, and evaluating service provided to cross cultural populations (opportunities and options have to be provided) (AAN, 1992, p. 281. Reprinted with permission.).

Diversity Among Nurses

Students complain that respect for cultural diversity is not applied to nurses. A student explains:

> The professors create this weird distinction that patients can have multicultural issues, but not nurses. That nurses are all the same. School reinforces that lesbians shouldn't be nurses. No one ever mentions that a patient may be gay or lesbian; and it's never, never true that a colleague may be gay or lesbian. There's no transfer from talking about patient differences to supporting differences among students.

A Cultural View of Nursing School

The limited pathophysiology oriented curriculum of most nursing schools makes sense when viewed from a cultural perspective. An instructor explains:

> The environment of nursing school doesn't honor diversity. The theme is that you treat everyone alike, from the perspective of white middle-class women. If you're someone else, you're never quite right, never quite good enough, you never quite fit in. In my opinion, you do more nursing if you treat everyone differently. Nursing education needs to address the issues of homophobia, sexism, racism, and able-bodyism rather than limiting what we consider to be nursing. These limitations stem from the bias of faculty members.

Another insightful faculty member says:

> I suspect that the weight in nursing curriculum around gay and lesbian issues is minuscule. The cultural component of patient care will be subordinated to the dominant value in nursing of diagnosing medical, surgical, and psychiatric disorders. We, as educators, have always had to submerge cultural issues. The issue of gay and lesbian cultural experience—even basic information—in an associate degree program can't be addressed because there are other priorities driven by issues of patient safety. Faculty is also not comfortable with gay issues. For them, it's the uncommon experience, the fearful experience. Faculty are unwilling to take the time, effort, or discomfort to learn about other cultures. Role modeling is a powerful teaching method. Faculty role model the dominant culture, and they value it. They can talk the talk of taking on the values of the client, but they can't do it.

A researcher agrees, "We socialize students into our profession in the most unhealthy and unthinking way: filling them full of facts, opinions, and procedures."

Concentrating on pathophysiology, rather than cultural issues, is supported by the state board exams. In many schools, the entire curriculum is geared to getting students to pass the exam. According to a spokesperson for the National Council of State Boards of Nursing, the group that designs the test, "The state board exam is a licensure test that measures entry-level minimum competence. The exam is interested in the care of the disease, not the person." In her eyes, culturally competent care is an advanced practice issue.

If that is true, then students should still expect their instructors, as advanced practitioners, to demonstrate culturally competent care in clinicals, even when cultural competence is excluded from classroom instruction because of time constraints. Only a few students reported this kind of practice being role modeled. Most instructors need remedial study to bring them up to the American Academy of Nursing's standards.

Curriculum

When asked if the health and emotional needs of lesbians and gay men were part of the curriculum at his college, an out professor responded, "In a word: No."

A woman who graduated last year remembers:

> Gay issues were not discussed, except briefly in psych. There was a one-page list of causes of gays and lesbians as pathology, such as poor bonding or childhood trauma. I demanded the psych instructor disclaim the information in class. She did, but the damage had already occurred. Several times, students made comments that gay men molest children. I felt an overwhelming sadness, real sadness, like crying. I don't argue in class, but I bring up the contradictory statement. I just can't let it go.

A gay man agrees, "All the development issues are assumed to be straight. That's sad. They don't consider us at all. Especially when you consider how hard it is to grow up to be gay. It makes me really mad."

When instructors try to incorporate gay and lesbian examples into class discussion, it may backfire because they either cannot disguise their biases, or are not sufficiently skilled to facilitate a discussion that questions students' values. One student was appalled when an instructor reinforced negative stereotypes about lesbians during a discussion that followed a video showing different kinds of birth experiences, including a lesbian couple. Instead of feeling included, she felt "scared and alienated."

Even in San Francisco, lesbian and gay issues are frequently ignored. A current student says:

> I'm still fuming from the peds class that described adolescent sexuality to the opposite gender as a developmental milestone. They later talked about gay adolescents in an almost marginalized way. They could have included gay adolescents as a part of growing up. To be more inclusive in simple ways, such as saying "sexual attraction" rather than "sexual attraction to the opposite gender."

Curricula neglect lesbian health issues. A lesbian student explains, "Instructors make an effort to include gay issues, but they mean gay men. Lesbians aren't included. They focus on AIDS." A lesbian instructor agrees, "The lesbian health content doesn't get the same respect. It's a leftover, last-minute thing. If it's a day-long conference, lesbians get a half hour."

Examples of Doing It Right

The best way to address gay and lesbian health issues is through examples. Separate classes on lesbian and gay health are not the answer. A nursing leader explains, "As with all issues, it should be part of the examples used in lectures. Using everyday examples and using critical thinking to apply to people who don't fit the stereotype."

A student describes a perfect example of integrating gay and lesbian issues into a clinical experience. "My maternity instructor said that last year a lesbian couple was treated badly, and that she was angry because the nursing staff was mean and terrible, an embarrassment. She said, 'I know that you students would never do that because you know better.'"

Another student proposes an overall strategy for including lesbian and gay issues, "In the minutiae of day-to-day things it has to change, but it would take just a small shift to make a difference to get information that's more useful, and make people feel less isolated." Another student asks that instructors "teach using the word *partner* instead of *husband.*"

Skillful instructors can expand examples to include social and emotional issues that may not be readily apparent to the novice student. An instructor explains, "AIDS has given me an opportunity to talk about gay people, including significant others and how oppression works. I'm in a unique position to talk about homophobia and how it works, but also how sexism works, and its economic consequences."

A student in San Francisco describes how an instructor demonstrated obtaining a history from a gay man. "One instructor who is gay brought in a man to interview. He role-modeled nonsexist, no-orientation language."

Instructors must also be skilled in dealing with the emotional reactions that lesbian and gay examples may engender. A gay student describes the aftermath of making a presentation about his volunteer work with AIDS patients to his psychology 101 class. "A couple of guys in the class made derogatory remarks, and I let the other students defend the issues. The instructor, not a nurse, was supportive and skilled. She handled the class as a group therapy session to deal with feelings and prejudices."

Another student describes a panel discussion with people who had been impacted by HIV. The panel included gay families, as well as traditional families. During another panel discussion, lesbian and gay people described their issues with health care.

LESBIAN AND GAY ROLE MODELS

Role models can be very influential, especially for students who are newly out. They demonstrate the normalcy of lesbian and gay people, and disprove the myth of invisibility. For all students, out instructors can set the tone that prejudiced remarks will not be tolerated. A gay instructor says, "Increasingly I don't feel content to be silent. I don't want students to have to wonder if they're in a safe environment. I feel a responsibility to the students."

But coming out for instructors can be almost as dangerous as it is for students. A tenured professor admits with sadness, "I want to be out so I can be a good role model, but I'm from the old school. I can't come out totally, not here. I'm proud of who and what I am, and what I've accomplished in life; and

I don't want to lose that security because of my sexual orientation. I would not have been as successful if I had come out
20 years ago."

Another instructor prides himself as an openly gay role
model, and has never had a negative experience as a result of
being out. "I say my partner this, or my friend that. I invite them
(gay and nongay students) over to my house for a pot luck at the
end of term so they can see that our lifestyle is OK."

He feels that openly lesbian and gay faculty can go the extra
mile for gay and lesbian students. He remembers, "One student
came to clinical after obviously sobbing, and he said he and his
lover had had a fight and the lover walked out. I told him to take
the day off and take care of his business. I wonder if a nongay
instructor could have been as empathetic." Respecting the
primacy of committed relationships is important to everyone, yet
lesbian and gay students rarely feel the safety to discuss their relationships or expect support.

A gay professor describes his style of being out:

> I talk about being gay in class. I would gladly come out at
> a faculty meeting. I'm out to the dean. We have an anti-
> discrimination clause, and that was important. Gay students
> and faculty will introduce themselves, but what they really
> want is to meet an out professor. I'm gradually growing into
> becoming a role model, because there are young people
> who want and need it. I feel the responsibility. I try to be
> there for them. I don't want to tell them not to be out, that
> they could get hurt, that they could get treated unfairly
> because of antigay sentiments. Instead, I try to nurture them.

Is there a price for being out? "Yes. There are some faculty
that limit their interaction with me. I don't know what I'm
missing, but they avoid me. It can result in poor communication.
I'm about 90% certain that my sexuality is the reason."

Another instructor is more selective in who she comes out to:

> I've had gay students, and I make a decision if they're
> sensible people who could be allies. If a student needs an
> ally, I come out to them. One gay man was convinced that
> he was the only one and was hated. He had been written
> up, and he needed support. I came out to him, and it might

have helped him personally, but he would have made it through school regardless.

An instructor described how being out helped when he had a difficult student. "A gay student flirted with me and wanted my home phone number, and I had to put limits. He was seductive by nature. My colleagues were supportive, and we assigned him to another clinical group." In another instance, a student sought him out for advice. "She was into shocking people, and she stepped on a lot of toes. I tried to help her sort out when it is appropriate to talk about issues."

A lesbian describes how most of her instructors functioned as role models, even when they did not reveal their sexual orientation. An important part of her development as a lesbian was leading a life free of the domination of men. "They provided a role model of women who were not involved with men. They were professional, skilled, and independent."

FIND A SUPPORTIVE SCHOOL

Selecting a supportive school is more difficult, yet more important, for lesbian and gay students. "If you're out and willing to broach the subject, and if you can relocate, I would encourage you to go to a school where you can blossom, rather than fight the tide of bigotry and hatred," says a gay nursing professor. "Fighting can drain a talented student."

If possible, strongly consider attending a college of nursing within a university, because the university may provide support. Moving away from home could also be a healthy choice for students who are newly coming out.

Assessing Nursing Schools

Assessing schools may be challenging for high school students who are inexperienced with lesbian and gay life, but it could prevent later problems. The needs of returning adult students are more diverse. Many approach school as a temporary job, and they do not expect much support. Other adult students seek an environment that supports their usual style of being out.

Assess the Community   The local lesbian and gay communities may be your greatest source of support.

▾ Read the local gay or feminist newspaper.

▾ Talk with someone at the lesbian or gay community center.

▾ Talk to a local student group or youth group that is not affiliated with a particular school.

▾ Is there a gay and lesbian hotline or helpline?

▾ Is there a local feminist or gay bookstore?

▾ Is there a local human rights ordinance or an ordinance sanctioning same-sex domestic partnerships?

Assess the University   For many students, the university may provide greater support for gays and lesbians than does the college of nursing.

▾ Talk to an admissions counselor.

▾ Check the list of student organizations to find a lesbian and gay support group.

▾ Read the student newspaper to find the local stand on lesbian and gay issues, as well as other "liberal" issues.

▾ Browse the gay or lesbian section in the university bookstore. If the section does not exist, it could be a bad sign.

▾ Look for the nondiscrimination statement in the student handbook. Does it include sexual orientation as a protected group?

▾ Does the university philosophy statement value diversity and respect exploration of individual differences?

▾ Check the student health service. How are issues of sexuality handled? Are there peer-support programs? How are gay and lesbian health issues handled? How are birth control issues handled? Solid support of heterosexual issues may also mean a healthy attitude toward lesbian and gay issues.

▾ If the university has a religious affiliation, does that preclude support for gay and lesbian organizations?

Assess the Nursing College or Department This may be the riskiest and most difficult assessment for students who do not wish to come out in the process. Students who wish to remain closeted can focus on cultural diversity or feminist issues and infer a similar climate for gay men and lesbians.

▾ Ask a faculty person to describe the climate.

▾ Talk with students, especially lesbians or gay men, about the climate.

▾ Ask a faculty person how issues of cultural and sexual diversity are handled.

▾ Is there cultural, racial, and gender diversity among the students and faculty?

▾ Do faculty research or publish about gay and lesbian health issues?

▾ How rigidly and stereotypically are gender roles expressed? Stereotyped thinking about gender and race usually spill over to sexual orientation as well.

SURVIVING A HOSTILE ENVIRONMENT

Sometimes students become trapped in a battle with a bigoted instructor, dean, or college. The student may be right, and the school wrong, but the school holds all the power. It may be too late to transfer to another school, and the student cares about nursing too much to quit. How do students survive without feeling that they are compromising their values? Unfortunately, this is the all-too-common position for gay and lesbian students.

Find a compassionate and savvy advisor. A lesbian instructor explains how she helps students:

> First, I try to validate the student's worth. At least in my office with the door shut, I can let them know that they're being treated unfairly, and acknowledge the pain. Usually

that requires a lot of listening on my part, and sometimes
tissues to wipe away the tears. But I also have to get them
to the place that they understand that being right isn't nearly
enough. We have to develop a strategy. Regardless of
pettiness, cruelty, and pain, they have to graduate.

A student, however, warns of seeking support from faculty
before you know them well. "Be very, very cautious about who
you come out to," she advises. "Be more than a little suspicious
about students and instructors who talk accepting. It can just be
lip service from a closeted right-wing conservative. Students are
vulnerable. It's harder to finish school at another place."

Some students lose their trust in school and look elsewhere
for support. A lesbian student concludes, "Realize that gay or
lesbian faculty may not be supportive of you even though they
should be your allies. They may fear reprisals if they are outed
or have to support gay or lesbian students."

Build Support

Successful students are able to build an informal coalition of
supporters from their classmates, faculty, friends, and people in
the lesbian and gay communities. "Identify allies and develop a
network of people who know and support you," advises a
student. "But don't look for school to provide that. Make it safe
for yourself by finding a pocket of people to support you."

Another student agrees, "Definitely make a bond with a
group that nurtures you as a wholesome person. Nursing school
is hard enough and bats you down. Find a community."

Almost all of the students interviewed found a small cadre
of classmates who supported them and enjoyed their company.
A gay man says, "The accepting and open-minded are the ones
I'm closest to. My friends accept it, and we joke about it."

Another student explains the need for support from her
classmates. "You need your nursing friends because they're the
only ones who can understand what it's like to watch a patient
die after she's extubated. But you can't share with them that you
spent last weekend in the mountains with your girlfriend."

Some students find their greatest support from each other.
"We helped each other to dream the big dream and believe that
this too shall pass," says a student. "We talked about how good

it would feel to tell somebody off. But in the end, we convinced each other not to blow up on the academic runway."

Many students also receive substantial support from their families. A young gay man says, "I'm out to my family and extended family, and they give me overwhelming support. My lover and I go to family functions together."

Support Groups

Schools that offer lesbian and gay support groups, usually outside the nursing school, can help. A student says, "The gay student's organization as a whole took a lot of pressure off me as an individual."

One student organized a support group within the college of nursing. "I ran a weekly lunch for gay and lesbian students. About seven showed up. Now it's sanctioned by the university. It's maybe one degree easier now to come out at school than before."

Some nursing students are reluctant to go to support groups. A lesbian faculty member says, "It's a great idea, but the nursing students are a little more concerned about the stigma, and they're in clinical so much that they don't avail themselves."

Survival Strategies

Even when you cannot change the environment, you can still determine how you are going to respond. Try these suggestions:

- ▾ Find a mentor or ally who is willing to wield influence on your behalf.

- ▾ Keep your ally informed of potential problems as early as possible to give you room to maneuver.

- ▾ Develop strategies with your ally. Practice the plan by role-modeling with your ally. Together devise a contingency plan, and agree on what events would initiate it. Provide your mentor with feedback about the outcome of each intervention. Winning plans are frequently shaped through trial and error.

- ▾ Share your feelings and frustrations with your ally. A true supporter will listen and validate your feelings to help reduce stress.

▾ Do not let your feelings spill over into class or clinical situations where they might harm you. Find a sympathetic listener away from school.

▾ If presented with vague complaints—such as "You just don't fit in here," or "Your attitude is unprofessional," or "I really like you as a person, but you don't seem to have what it takes to be a nurse"—in a firm but controlled fashion, redirect the issue to concrete measurable behaviors. Ask for specific examples. In essence ask, "What exactly do you expect me to do?" Ask for a time line. If necessary, develop written contracts. All instructors are expected to provide objectives, and all students are entitled to feedback. Sometimes it is more powerful to let your mentor negotiate these behavioral objectives and time lines.

▾ Before you enroll in a class, screen the instructor. Nurses love to gossip; use it to your advantage.

▾ If necessary, interview the instructor before signing up for the class. Ask, "What do you expect? How do you like to work with students? This is who I am, do you think we would be happy working together?"

▾ If damage occurs, control it. Avoid the thrill of turning any single incident into a catastrophe.

▾ Keep your sense of humor.

▾ Maintain a rich and full life away from school. Indulge yourself in safe pleasures. Find a haven within the gay and lesbian communities.

▾ Remember that nothing goads a bigot more than your success.

SUMMARY

For lesbian and gay students, most nursing schools exaggerate the prejudices and discrimination experienced in other walks of life. Despite paying lip service to cultural diversity, nursing schools continue to perpetuate the myth that nurses are all white, middle-class, heterosexual women. The current predominance of white female nurses speaks for itself.

Most nursing schools fail to meet the basic emotional needs of gay and lesbian students, especially younger students. If nursing schools were not such hostile places for lesbian and gay students, more of them would be out. Nursing schools also fail by perpetuating the myth of invisibility. Schools graduate practitioners unskilled and unaccustomed to providing care in an inclusive fashion.

But students bring hope. They recognize that they are enduring a prejudiced system that is far more restrictive than the other parts of their life. Over the past 25 years, the trend has been to come out. Compared to earlier generations of lesbian and gay people, tomorrow's young students will spend less time questioning whether they should come out, and more time questioning the competence of the bigots who discriminate against them. The same is true for returning adult students who are secure in their identity. Nursing schools will have to remedy their prejudices in order to prepare for tomorrow's students.

The other hope comes from isolated schools where faculty members have risked coming out, or have in other quieter ways improved the climate for diversity. Their struggle is heroic. For example, the commencement address in 1994 for the combined degree program of Lienhard School of Nursing, Pace University was delivered by an out gay man. Pace recruits a diverse student body into nursing. Almost 20% of the class were men, the average age was 34 years, and students came from six foreign countries. He said in part:

> We have found . . . that our diversity has helped us, both in our studies and in our student practice. We bring our whole selves into nursing, and use over 600 years of life experience as a reason why employers should hire us. Perhaps that is the most important lesson that we have learned here at Pace; that our diverse experiences, our opinions—and we do have opinions—and our very differences are our greatest strength. Together with our technical preparation, it is our diversity that uniquely empowers us to care for clients who are even more diverse than we are. (Reprinted with permission of the speaker.)

References

American Academy of Nursing Expert Panel on Culturally Competent Nursing Care. (1992). AAN expert panel report: Culturally competent health care. *Nursing Outlook, 40*(6), 277–283.

Bennett, M. J. (1986). A developmental approach to training for intercultural sensitivity. *International Journal of Intercultural Relations, 10,* 179–196.

Cass, V. C. (1979). Homosexual identity formation: A theoretical model. *Journal of Homosexuality, 4*(3), 219–235.

Duncan, D. (1990). Prevalence of sexual assault victimization among heterosexual and gay/lesbian university students. *Psychological Reports, 66*(1), 65–66.

Eliason, M. J., & Randall, C. E. (1991). Lesbian phobia in nursing students. *Western Journal of Nursing Research, 13*(3), 363–374.

Eliason, M., Donelan, C., & Randall, C. (1992). Lesbian stereotypes. *Health Care for Women International, 13*(2), 131–144.

Herek, G. M. (1993). Documenting prejudice against lesbians and gay men on campus: The Yale sexual orientation survey. *Journal of Homosexuality, 25*(4), 15–30.

Randall, C. E. (1989). Lesbian phobia among BSN educators: A survey. *Journal of Nursing Education, 28*(7), 302–305.

Stephany, T. M. (1992). Faculty support for gay and lesbian nursing students. *Nurse Educator, 17*(5), 22–23.

8 | ORGANIZED NURSING'S RESPONSE

Stand up for your human rights. Insist on being treated like a person, not some sort of dysfunctional anomaly.

A lesbian nurse

First off, whether you're gay or straight, nurses don't band together and support one another. When you see someone else who is out and having trouble, support them. It's gutsy, but you have to do it. Support them professionally first, then emotionally.

A lesbian staff nurse in the South

BASIC ISSUES

Although there is wide diversity within the many gay and lesbian communities, there is also general agreement on fundamental issues. In order to respect the basic needs of lesbian and gay nurses, the following issues need to be considered:

- ▾ End discrimination at work and at school.
- ▾ Honor the historic achievements of lesbian and gay nurses.

▾ Ensure that gay and lesbian clients receive culturally competent and prejudice-free care.

▾ Encourage and support professional publications concerning lesbian and gay clients and nurses.

▾ Encourage and support research concerning gay and lesbian clients, nurses, and the effects of nurses' attitudes on care.

▾ Bring benefits and employee assistance programs for lesbian and gay nurses and their partners into parity with those already enjoyed by other nurses.

▾ Encourage and support affinity groups for gay and lesbian nurses.

END DISCRIMINATION

In its bylaws, the American Nurses Association (ANA) includes sexual orientation as a class protected from discrimination, and state nurses associations follow ANA's lead. The association also encourages similar antidiscrimination language in the contracts state associations negotiate; and inclusion of sexual orientation no longer raises objections, according to an ANA spokesperson.

"More importantly," says an insider, "the ANA role-models nondiscrimination among its members. This is a very supportive atmosphere for gays and lesbians to take leadership, and gay and lesbian people are significantly represented."

The gay and lesbian caucus of the House of Delegates meets informally during the ANA's conventions and determines how and when to raise issues. Members of the caucus are especially proud of the leadership they have taken in AIDS issues and the issue of discrimination against lesbians and gay men in the military.

ANA Code of Ethics

The most powerful statement in ANA's *Code for Nurses with Interpretive Statements* (last modified in 1985) comes in the opening precept: "The nurse provides service with respect for human dignity and the uniqueness of the client, unrestricted by considerations of social or economic status, personal attributes, or the nature of health problems." Of the many paragraphs interpreting this statement, three sentences are most telling:

- ▼ "The fundamental principle of nursing practice is respect for the inherent dignity and worth of every client."

- ▼ "The need for health care is universal, transcending all national, ethnic, racial, religious, political, educational, economic, developmental, personality, role, and sexual differences."

- ▼ "The nurse's concern for human dignity and the provision of high-quality nursing care is not limited by personal attitudes or beliefs."

These statements are honorable but ambiguous in relation to sexual orientation. Why does the list in the second sentence quoted use very specific terms to define most groups, but use the ambiguous term *sexual differences*? Does it mean gender, sexual orientation, or both?

State Nurses Associations

Because ANA is really a federation of state and local associations, political action occurs most appropriately at the state level. A casual survey of state associations reveals a wide variety of responses to lesbian and gay issues. The California Nurses Association, for example, can clearly articulate its stand and refer nurses to district-sanctioned affinity groups for lesbian and gay nurses. Most state associations are very small and unaware of gay and lesbian issues. Responses on the telephone include: "Oh, don't tell me that they're a group that's discriminated against too!" or "None of our members raise these issues" or "We do whatever ANA tells us to do in terms of discrimination."

However, the receptionist at a small state association gave a very specific answer. One of the board members is an out gay man, and the receptionist offered his telephone number for help and support. This could be the answer from every receptionist if lesbian and gay nurse leaders came out. State associations respond to the needs of their members. It is up to gay and lesbian nurses to raise issues locally. As one student observes, "By not coming out, you tacitly endorse the stereotype. It is unrealistic to expect other people to raise consciousness for us."

End Discrimination in the Military

California and at least two other state associations passed resolutions forcing disclaimers in its advertising clarifying that the military discriminates against gay and lesbian nurses in contrast with the state association's policy of not discriminating. As a result, the military stopped advertising in the California state association newspaper, a substantial loss of revenue.

On the national level, the ANA endorsed a similar ban on military advertising in *The American Nurse*, a decision that could translate into $80,000 in lost revenue. The ban is scheduled to go into effect in 1996; but insiders predict a battle that will delay implementation.

The ANA has consistently supported Colonel Margarethe Cammermeyer, a lesbian nurse who won an appeal in federal appeals court to be reinstated as the Chief Nurse of the Washington state National Guard. She had been discharged after admitting to being a lesbian. In 1994, ANA awarded her its human rights award.

Censure Discriminatory Behavior

Currently few lesbian or gay nurses or students know how to address their grievances if they become victims of discrimination. The nursing profession provides little information about fighting antigay discrimination. Nor does it actively censure nurses or institutions that discriminate against lesbian and gay nurses, students, or patients.

Who monitors complaints from gay and lesbian students about discrimination by their instructors? Who questions the accreditation of nursing schools that demonstrate a pattern of discrimination? Who tells narrow-minded nursing students, certain that they could never treat a lesbian or gay man, that they cannot ethically function as professional nurses?

The same questions could be asked about health care organizations and individual nurses. If nurses follow the ANA Code of Ethics, why does nursing tolerate bigotry among its practitioners, schools, and employers?

A National Statement

Nursing as a profession is guilty of not stating a clear policy about gay men and lesbians. Couching the issue in the language of universal human dignity dilutes and confuses the message, and it contributes to the myth that lesbians and gay men do not exist.

Because there are so few men and racial minorities in nursing, lesbians and gays are in fact the largest minority group. There are almost twice as many lesbian nurses than there are either African-American or Latino nurses. Nursing associations meet the needs of their members by addressing gay and lesbian issues.

Nursing is far behind other helping professions in publicly supporting lesbians and gay men. In 1973, the American Psychiatric Association removed homosexuality from its official list of mental disorders; and in 1975, the American Psychological Association adopted a resolution: "Homosexuality, per se, implies no impairment in judgment, stability, reliability, or general social or vocational capabilities. Further the APA urges all mental health professionals to take the lead in removing the stigma of mental illness that has long been associated with homosexual orientations" (American Psychological Association, 1991). Even the conservative American Medical Association recently adopted a policy that, according to a spokesperson, calls for "nonjudgmental recognition of sexual orientation."

The National Association of Social Workers (NASW) provides a model of the kind of statement that nursing could adopt. The "National Association of Social Workers Code of Ethics" (1994) includes sexual orientation in its nondiscrimination statements concerning the social worker's ethical responsibility to clients.

The code also guides social workers to "act to prevent practices that are inhumane or discriminatory . . . [including] . . . employment policies and practices."

In the preamble to its full policy statement on gay and lesbian issues, the NASW makes the connection between practitioners' prejudices and the quality of care they deliver: "Prejudice toward lesbian and gay people and discomfort about social work

practice with this population may lead to inappropriate, ineffec-
tive, and even damaging interventions by social workers" (p. 163).
Is this not also true of nurses' prejudices? The policy outlines specific efforts related to education, antidiscrimination, public awareness, health and mental health services, and legal and political
action. The complete policy is included in Appendix B.

To monitor gay and lesbian issues, state chapters of the
national association form interest groups. For example, the
Illinois chapter formed the Lesbian and Gay Social Work Network
for practitioners, educators, and students. The Network identifies
practice issues, develops resources, and recommends practice
standards and policies. The group also monitors gay and lesbian
issues in school curricula and field work placements.

If social workers can outline concrete measures to combat
discrimination, why can't nursing?

Support Coming Out

Stigma and discrimination make it more difficult to come out and
create a cascade of events that result in poor emotional and physical health for lesbians and gay men. HIV disease is an obvious
example. Richard Ferri, RN, PhD, ANP, president of the
Association of Nurses in AIDS Care says:

> There is a rebirth of discrimination against gay and lesbian
> people that is gaining momentum and support. It drives
> people back into the closet, reduces their self-esteem; and
> as a result, there is a real potential to increase the number
> of people who will get infected with HIV. Gay men are still
> the largest group of people in the AIDS epidemic. We need
> to go back and address the needs of gay adolescents and
> young gay men. We need to role-model healthy gay and
> lesbian images, not just role-model safe sex. We cannot
> tolerate bigotry. We must support coming out.

Discrimination prevents gay and lesbian nurses from acting
as healthy role models and prevents lesbian and gay clients from
finding helpful partners in their health care. It delivers the message that gay and lesbian people and their health are unimpor-
tant. Discrimination   and   the   closet   it   builds   support

self-destructive health behaviors. Ferri's observation of the link between the closet and HIV infection also applies to cancer, chemical dependence, and any disease that requires early detection, a high degree of patient adherence to therapy, or long-term management.

Supporting coming out promotes positive lesbian and gay role models and says to clients: As a gay or lesbian person, you are important and taking care of yourself is an expression of the high esteem in which you are held.

The National Association of Social Workers (NASW) statement on Gay and Lesbian Issues (1993) states in part: "Social workers and the social work profession can support and empower lesbian and gay people through all phases of the coming out process." For the sake of our patient's mental and physical health, nurses must also support and empower coming out. Appendix B contains the full NASW statement.

HONOR THE HISTORY OF LESBIAN AND GAY NURSES

"No one will ever know that the academic discipline of nursing was founded and nurtured by lesbians, because these women weren't out," says a young gay academic. "Most of the great nursing leaders at least through the 1970s were lesbians. Most were deeply closeted."

A nurse historian, who chose to remain anonymous, agrees in principle, "A great number of nurses who were closeted lesbians have made significant contributions to nursing and that includes some of the early leaders. We haven't talked about them." It is, however, difficult to define lesbian relationships during the Victorian era when gay and lesbian affection was also known as the "love that dare not speak its name." She explains, "There's no absolute documentation. We can infer from letters that a relationship was close and involved love. But does that mean sisterly affection or physical love? I would surmise that some were lesbians, but I can't prove it."

Florence Nightingale once wrote: "I have lived and slept in the same bed with English countesses and Prussian farm women

. . . no woman has excited passions among women more than I have" (Alyson, 1989).

The real issue is not scholarship, but stigma. Too many nurses assume that discussing whether Florence Nightingale, for example, might have been a lesbian would only drag her through the mud and serve no real purpose. This denies lesbian and gay nurses and especially nursing students access to historic role models. Politely ignoring the question of sexual orientation has robbed gay and lesbian nurses of their past and perpetuates the myth of invisibility.

A nurse who has sought out her lesbian foremothers explains, "It made a difference to me that early nursing thought was tied to lesbianism. They tell me that it's OK to be a lesbian nurse. I have something in common with great nurses."

Acknowledging the sexual orientation of our historic nursing leaders tells young gay and lesbian nurses: You too can make a contribution and succeed. It is time to bring the past accomplishments of lesbian and gay nurses out of the shadow of prejudice and into the light of scholarship. "It's well overdue to talk about this," concludes the historian.

ENSURE CULTURALLY COMPETENT CARE

Nursing supports culturally competent care, but few practitioners realize that it also applies to lesbians and gay men. "Culturally competent care is defined as care that is sensitive to issues related to culture, race, gender, and sexual orientation, provided within the cultural context of the client," says Marilyn Douglas, RN, DNSc, CCRN, the president of the Transcultural Nursing Society. "Although we (the Transcultural Nursing Society) don't have an official position, we support, in spirit, that sexual orientation is considered a culture in itself; and therefore, culturally competent care is required."

This echoes the 1992 statement from the American Academy of Nursing Expert Panel on Culturally Competent Nursing Care: "In addition, there are minority populations that have received limited attention in the health care system, and they need to be considered and included. Examples are gay and lesbian populations . . . " (AAN, 1992, p. 278).

The panel also addresses the need for more information about gay men and lesbians: "There is limited information on and knowledge about values, beliefs, experiences, and health care needs of some of these populations, such as lesbians, gays, and immigrants" (AAN, 1992, p. 278). The panel recommends continued research, development of care models based on cultural competence, and education.

The National League for Nursing also supports culturally competent care. "Throughout the history of the NLN, the issue of cultural diversity has always been important," says a spokesperson. "The NLN encourages the discussion of lesbian and gay issues." However, the League has not yet identified specific issues, nor has it included these issues in specific accreditation standards.

Culturally competent care is not a luxury, but the basic need of gay and lesbian clients. "We've ignored the cultural aspects of why a gay man might not seek health care because of a provider who is so entrenched in heterosexism," says a national leader in lesbian and gay health care. "We don't exist. There is no appropriate language to describe our relationships. Gay and lesbian clients get short shrift because no one asks the right questions or makes a safe environment. Gay clients need to have partners included in patient teaching to improve compliance."

Other helping professions are ahead of nursing in identifying the specific issues of providing sensitive care for lesbian and gay clients. "Social workers and counselors are expected by their national organizations to be proficient in dealing with gay and lesbian people," says a gay educator. "No such standard exists for nursing. I think a call on the national level would cause a stir."

Acknowledge the Full Range of Health Issues

For too many people, being gay is synonymous with being a man, and lesbians are excluded. Being gay is also synonymous with being infected with HIV. "We have translated being gay into having AIDS, when it comes to organized nursing," says a nurse caring for lesbian and gay patients. A staffer at ANA agrees, "Outside of AIDS, we have not been as aggressive about teaching nursing about gay and lesbian issues."

The most significant issue that affects both women and men is access to culturally competent care. Some practitioners actively discriminate against lesbians and gay men, but a greater number of practitioners humiliate patients with questions such as "Who plays the part of the man?" or they ask questions for which gay and lesbian people cannot give a brief, reasonable answer. How does a lesbian in a long-term relationship answer the question "Are you married?" or "Are you having sexual intercourse?"

How can lesbian and gay patients trust practitioners who cannot even ask the simple questions correctly? For many people, the solution is to ignore routine health care and only seek episodic, emergency care when they cannot wait any longer. How many tumors could have been detected early or strokes avoided if the practitioner had provided gay- and lesbian-sensitive care that developed a relationship with the real person who was the patient? How many patients do not follow the prescribed course of treatment because their partner was not part of the patient education or the plan of care?

Even when lesbian and gay patients find sensitive outpatient care, it rarely leads to sensitive inpatient care. Standardized hospital forms almost never acknowledge the possibility of a gay or lesbian person. If patients are treated badly, their partners are treated even worse. They are usually expected to be invisible—to only visit during general visiting hours, not ask the nurse any questions, and not have an opinion about how to care for their loved ones.

Use Language that Avoids Bias

One part of the solution to providing culturally competent care is to avoid the automatic assumption that all patients and nurses are heterosexual. Appendix C contains suggestions to avoid heterosexual bias in language developed by the Committee on Lesbian and Gay Concerns of the American Psychological Association. These suggestions are not, however, guidelines adopted by the APA.

Using these suggestions could prevent the heterosexist tone in hospital forms and in nursing publications. They could also help nursing instructors to discuss patient cases in a way that includes everyone. Most nursing publications already purport to follow APA guidelines. Including these suggestions to avoid heterosexual bias would extend the scope and depth of nursing publications.

Encourage Publications

Publishers are reluctant to illustrate common health concerns by using lesbian or gay patients. Instead, examples are restricted to HIV disease, depression or suicide, and chemical dependency.

One author quarreled with an editor over keeping a lesbian example in an article about training. Eventually she withdrew the manuscript, and she suspects the editor feared appearing to be a lesbian by citing lesbian examples.

Frequently, articles about gay and lesbian issues are published in journals with limited circulation that may not be available in hospital libraries. In Chicago, for example, the *Journal of Homosexuality* is not available in the medical libraries of most major hospitals, and it is found in only a few university libraries. The *Journal of Transcultural Nursing* suffers the same limited availability.

The solution is to mainstream lesbian and gay examples into articles about common diseases written for journals with wider circulation. Why not include a gay man as an example of a patient with a broken arm? Or describe a lesbian who has had a myocardial infarction in a discussion of adherence to medical treatment? What role would her partner have in the outcome of the patient's treatment? Or include gay and lesbian adolescents in articles about growth and development?

Nurses can improve the image of lesbians and gay men in print and increase the amount of coverage. On a local level, suggest gay- and lesbian-sensitive books for your hospital or school medical library. Become a media watchdog. Write letters to the journal editors to provide feedback about the missed opportunities to include lesbian or gay patient examples or to correct misleading information. Let the editor know that gay and lesbian health issues extend far beyond HIV disease. Currently, a lot is written about cultural competence, but almost none of it includes lesbian or gay examples.

SUPPORT RESEARCH

Aside from AIDS and chemical dependency, there has been little nursing research concerning lesbian and gay health care issues. Says one researcher, "People were very nervous about my researching nurse educators, especially talking about our biases."

Several graduate students and doctoral candidates who wanted to explore lesbian or gay issues told the same story. Their instructors questioned the value of the project; their advisors insisted that faculty were not qualified to form a committee; their classmates giggled or made derisive comments instead of offering valuable criticism; their dean insisted that there were not enough research subjects to make the research possible. Invariably the project—regardless of its scientific merits—emitted a political odor. Closeted faculty felt threatened and shunned the project altogether, and even well-grounded faculty questioned whether they wanted to go to bat over a politically and emotionally charged issue. The end result: Another valuable project sabotaged by fear, ignorance, and prejudice. The surprise is not that there is so little research about gay and lesbian issues, but that there is any at all.

One solution might be establishment of research fellowships or funds earmarked to support research into lesbian and gay health issues. For example, 10% of total research awards could be designated for gay and lesbian research. These issues could be piggybacked onto other projects.

To remove bias, all nursing researchers should increase the cultural sensitivity of their work. Researchers need to identify their own cultural biases and incorporate cultural awareness into their studies (Henderson, Sampselle, Mayes, & Oakley, 1992). The myth that all people are heterosexuals pervades many research questions and methodologies. Heterosexual bias must be removed from research questions and questionnaires.

BENEFITS FOR DOMESTIC PARTNERS

According to an ANA spokesperson, the association encourages negotiators to bargain for benefits for domestic partners, and its own contract with employees includes these benefits. The issue is usually determined by dollars, not discrimination. "Regardless of whether the director of nursing who sits across the negotiating table is gay or straight," says a seasoned nurse negotiator, "the arguments against domestic partner benefits are economic. But it seems easier when someone on the management side is gay."

Although health care benefits for same-sex domestic partners are becoming more widely available, benefits need to be extended to create parity with heterosexual married people. Chapter 5 includes suggestions for organizing support for benefits for same-sex domestic partners. For more information, see *Pride at Work: Organizing for Lesbian and Gay Rights in Unions* by Miriam Frank and Desma Holcomb and the Lesbian and Gay Labor Network of New York, P.O. Box 1159, Peter Stuyvesant Station, New York, NY 10009.

EMPLOYEE ASSISTANCE PROGRAMS

Lesbian and gay employees are entitled to the same range of resources available to heterosexual employees through employee assistance programs. For example, nurses with relationship problems should have access to gay- and lesbian-sensitive counseling in the same way that mixed-gender couples have access to marriage counseling.

Nurses with chemical dependency issues are entitled to access to sensitive counseling and drug rehabilitation programs. State nurses associations that act as referral sources for impaired nurses must maintain referrals for lesbian- and gay-sensitive counselors.

Nurses and nursing students who need support when coming out are entitled to referrals to local lesbian and gay community services, as well as access to counselors who are experienced with coming out issues. Nurses victimized by discrimination may also need access to confidential counseling and advice with grievance procedures. Employers could establish a liaison office within their human resources department to coordinate services and referrals for gay and lesbian employees.

LESBIAN AND GAY AFFINITY GROUPS

Many nurses seek support groups. "I just want to know that there are other people out there with the same issues," says a nurse in a rural area. "It could be an outlet to get feedback, support, and help with problem solving. I want to be able to bounce things off people, and to share the joys."

Nurses in some areas meet locally to gain support, work on political issues, or enjoy social camaraderie. To find a group in your area, call your local nurses association or look for ads in the gay and lesbian or alternative press. Sometimes information is only passed by word of mouth.

Organizing Affinity Groups

The Alameda County Nurses Association, Lesbian Nurses Interest Group is an example of an officially sanctioned group. Sponsored by a local district of the California Nurses Association, the group advertises at no expense in the local nurses association newsletter. The group started in 1989 as a gay and lesbian group, but no men came to the meetings. At the first meeting, which attracted about 30 nurses, the group decided not to be anonymous, and as a result about half of the nurses did not return.

According to Chris, one of the founders, the group evolved from building internal support, to political activism, to ongoing social support. In the beginning, they worked to develop a shared direction. They discussed coming out issues, who they were as individual nurses, and what they wanted from an organization. Chris cites the political work as a way to help the group grow through a shared purpose. They marched in the Gay and Lesbian Day Parade, advocated for a disclaimer concerning discrimination in advertisements to recruit military nurses, and wrote articles for the local nursing press. At the ANA convention, they hosted a hospitality suite for the gay and lesbian caucus (Stephany, 1992).

Other groups combine health care workers from different professions to make the group more viable. They find many commonalities around lesbian and gay issues despite the differences in their professional backgrounds.

If you are planning to start an affinity group, consider the following questions:

- ▼ Where will you meet? Does your employer, nurses association, or lesbian or gay organization offer low-cost or free space? If you decide to meet in a home, will it always be in the same house, or will it rotate among members?

- ▼ Does your local nurses association or gay or lesbian community center offer technical assistance in running groups or maintaining mailing lists?

- ▼ Will the group be open to new members on an ongoing basis, or will membership be restricted to a negotiated series of meetings?

- ▼ What is the intended membership: men, women, students, nurses only, or all health care workers?

- ▼ Is it possible for members to attend anonymously, or will you keep mailing lists?

- ▼ If you advertise, will you list the time and location of the meeting, or have potential members call for details? Will callers be assured confidentiality?

Cassandra

From 1982 to 1988, the group Cassandra offered a radical feminist viewpoint to nursing. The organization was named after the figure in Greek mythology who was loved by the god Apollo and was granted the power to predict the future. When she spurned his love, the jealous Apollo twisted her gifts. Although she could still predict the future, no one believed her prophecies. The name perfectly fit the group's politics.

Peggy Chinn, RN, PhD, FAAN, editor of *Advances in Nursing Science*, and one of the group's founders, explains: "The purpose was to raise consciousness by applying a feminist analysis to issues of nursing. We specifically wanted a radical feminist analysis." Although the group was not exclusively for lesbians, it was supportive of open lesbians.

They published a newsletter entitled *Cassandra: Radical Feminist Nurses Newsjournal* and sponsored annual gatherings that combined consciousness raising, networking, and women's music. In 1984, they sparked controversy at the ANA convention by giving a presentation. Because some nurses were offended and did not want to acknowledge lesbians, Cassandra was excluded from future conventions.

Eventually, the group dissolved due to the rift between open lesbians, closeted lesbians, lesbian-supportive heterosexuals, and heterosexual women who were edgy about associating with lesbians. One long-term member recalls, "Cassandra drove a lot of closeted lesbians underground. There was also dissent from nonlesbians about whether Cassandra was really a lesbian organization or a feminist organization. They couldn't see a common purpose."

The Gay Nurses' Alliance

The Gay Nurses' Alliance (GNA) came out at the 1973 Pennsylvania State Nurses Association annual convention with an unsanctioned, but well-received, educational exhibit. The original founders, E. Carolyn Innes and David Waldron, pushed for national recognition the following year at the ANA convention, where they exhibited, hosted a hospitality suite, and made a two-hour presentation entitled "Gay People: Straight Health Care" to a packed audience.

Two years later, Waldron was appointed to ANA's newly established Commission on Human Rights. In 1978, the ANA passed a resolution sponsored by the commission that "supports the enactment of civil rights laws at the local, state, and federal levels which would provide the same protection to persons regardless of sexual and affectional preference as it is currently guaranteed to others on the basis of sex, age, ethnicity, and color."

GNA continued to exhibit at ANA conventions, and early members wrote articles about gay and lesbian issues for nursing journals. In its heyday, approximately 300 women and men joined the national organization, and many also participated in local chapters.

According to a flyer ("Current Goals," undated) produced by the organization in the 1970s, the group's goals included:

▾ To provide a forum where gay nurses can talk together.

▾ To foster an awareness that gay people exist both as patients and members of the nursing profession.

▾ To provide information to refute stereotypes about gay people.

▾ To aid nurses who experience job discrimination because they are gay.

▾ To improve the quality of care gay patients receive.

▾ To diagnose and treat homophobia.

"Gay and lesbian nurses were empowered to raise issues and make changes in their hospitals or state nurses associations," says a former member. "People came to the annual meetings and felt empowered, but also shocked that they weren't the only ones. They lacked role models who admitted that they're happy to be gay."

Today GNA is inactive. "A lot of the history of the Gay Nurses Alliance is erased because the people died," says a former member. "It's gone forever. It slipped away in the late eighties because of AIDS."

LOST GROUND DUE TO AIDS

It is impossible to overestimate the amount of potential progress that has been lost in the struggle for civil rights for gay men and lesbians because of AIDS. "A lot of our leaders both within nursing and in the gay community have died of AIDS," says a gay man. Unfortunately, the wave of deaths has not yet stopped. "It's tough to mentor because the people you're mentoring also die of AIDS," he says.

How will the next generation of lesbian and gay leaders learn the skills they need to move forward? The heavy loss of gay men has caused a separation with even the near past. Because of the poor recording of gay and lesbian history, the community relies on oral tradition. Now a group of elders is missing. Fewer people are available to pass on a vision, as well as strategies of how to wage the battle for human rights.

Many lesbian and gay nurses have heroically shouldered the responsibility of caring for people with AIDS, pushing for humane treatment for people with AIDS, and teaching the profession how to respond to the epidemic. But this valiant effort has left fewer resources available to continue to push for other gay and lesbian professional issues.

SUMMARY

As a profession, nursing has responded well to support people with HIV disease. Now it is time to extend that support to all gay men and lesbians. Nursing is far behind other helping professions in offering support. As the largest minority group within nursing, lesbian and gay nurses deserve the support of their professional organizations. Nursing needs to clarify its position concerning gay and lesbian patients and nurses in a unified, unambiguous way. It is no longer enough to expect lesbians and gay men to melt into the language of universal human dignity, and thus seem invisible. The profession also needs to police its members and schools to put an end to bigotry.

References

Alyson Publications. (1989). *The Alyson almanac.* Boston: Author.

American Academy of Nursing Expert Panel on Culturally Competent Nursing Care. (1992). AAN expert panel report: Culturally competent health care. *Nursing Outlook, 40*(6), 277–283.

American Nurses Association. (1985). *Code for nurses with interpretive statements.* Washington, DC: American Nurses Publishing.

American Psychological Association. Committee on Lesbian and Gay Concerns. (1991). *American Psychological Association policy statements on lesbian and gay concerns.* Washington, DC: Author.

American Psychological Association. Committee on Lesbian and Gay Concerns. (1991). Avoiding heterosexual bias in language. *American Psychologist, 46*(9), 973–974.

Current Goals of GNA. (undated). The Gay Nurses' Alliance. (Information provided by the Gay and Lesbian Historical Society of Northern California, San Francisco, CA.)

Henderson, D. J., Sampselle, C., Mayes, F., & Oakley, D. (1992). Toward culturally sensitive research in a multicultural society. *Health Care for Women International, 13*(2), 339–350.

National Association of Social Workers. (1994). Lesbian and gay issues. *Social Work Speaks,* 3rd edition, pp. 162–165.

Stephany, T. M. (1992). Promoting mental health: Lesbian nurse support groups. *Journal of Psychosocial Nursing, 30*(20), 35–38.

9 | HOW HIGH THE LAVENDER CEILING?

I made a decision that I need to be out. I was getting sick in the closet. What effect it will have on my nursing career, I don't know. It could create opportunities, or it could restrict opportunities.

A lesbian nurse

This is not the time for survival. We're too comfortable. If you just want to survive your shift or get your promotion, then stay in the closet. Always push for inclusion, even in the smallest ways. Is sexual orientation included in your hospital's policies or forms? If not, then make it a point to say: You left me out, I'm sure you didn't intend to.

A gay nurse practitioner

NURSES FEEL A CEILING

Many gay and lesbian nurses recognize the price for being out—staying at the bedside or in low-level management positions. A lesbian staff nurse says, "There's definitely a ceiling. If you're gay or lesbian, and you want to be an assistant nurse manager, that's

OK, but not a nurse manager, regardless of how good you are." She bases her opinion on experience. "Despite high morale, low turnover, and little sick time, a gay man filling a temporary nurse manager position was turned down for the promotion. Instead they hired an inept straight nurse."

Another nurse agrees, "I don't care if you have a PhD or six master's degrees, you're not going to get to the executive offices, regardless of how well versed you are. You can be a worker, but not a chieftain."

Lesbians and gay men are more vulnerable to discrimination because of the wide variation in legal protection. For many employers, it is perfectly legal to discriminate. A lesbian says, "Unfortunately, it's too much at the whim of your boss."

A gay man who served for 11 years as a vice director says, "The trend is getting worse as the country is getting more Republican, more conservative, more religious right. Here the hospital CEO pressured the director of nursing to get rid of gays."

This chapter examines the dynamics of the lavender ceiling—the colliding influences of gender, age, sexual orientation, individual prejudices, and corporate culture.

ROLE MODELS

Openly lesbian and gay role models in leadership positions give concrete proof that gay men and lesbians can succeed. A gay nurse beginning his career and hoping to move up the administrative ladder says lesbian and gay nurses can succeed because "the dean of my undergrad nursing program and the director of nursing at my first hospital were both gay."

Another nurse agrees, "I had a friend who was a director. It was unspoken that she was a lesbian, and she had no problems. I don't feel that I would have problems if I wanted to work up the ladder."

A nurse manager describes an institutional climate that fosters lesbian and gay role models. "There are so many gay and lesbian people at this hospital that it's almost the norm. Because there's a gay supervisor, a VP, and a head nurse, it feels safe." She accounts for the climate in part because the staff is young and well-educated. Its university affiliation fosters liberal policies including protection from discrimination and a cultural diversity program.

A young man who just graduated from nursing school says, "It's important that successful nurses come out so that everyone knows that gay and lesbian people make a contribution."

The Lavender Network

The gay and lesbian communities provide information networks for insiders. "I have known some gay women leaders, who I wouldn't otherwise have known, and they have helped me," says a volunteer leader with recent experience in more than one national nursing organization. "There's an old gay girls' network. You can call people across the country and tap that resource for the rest of your life."

People outside the community may know that it exists, but not how to access it. A graduate student says, "Some straight nurses complain about the lavender network: Everybody knows everybody, and they feel left out."

DIFFERENCES BETWEEN MEN AND WOMEN?

Stereotypes based on gender and sexual orientation sometimes clash. On one hand, men are stereotyped as leaders. A gay man says, "As a man, there's a push toward management and leadership." Women often feel discriminated against first as women. "My director of nursing is pretty closed minded," says a lesbian nurse. "For her, if you don't have a penis, you're not worth anything."

On the other hand, women seem to hide their sexual orientation more easily than can men. A lesbian says, "For lesbians, there's less discrimination because men can't imagine that a woman could survive without a man. So they don't assume that you're a lesbian." A gay man agrees, "It becomes very political when you climb the ladder, especially for men. It's different for women, they can pass it off easier."

However, women who are identified as lesbians may suffer more discrimination than do men. "It's sad, but I'd tell women to be closeted, and men to come out," says a lesbian. "Women are not threatened by gay men. Straight women are afraid that lesbians will come on to them, or they'll be labeled a lesbian by association."

A staff nurse puts it in perspective, "It's easier for women to hide, especially for me because I have a child. People in the South think that lesbians are much rarer, but more shocking. They think that lesbians are exotic and bizarre."

A lesbian executive agrees, "I'll bet you that it's much harder for men than for women. Women must go much farther to be an in-your-face lesbian. They don't want a gay woman at the top, but I bet it's harder to be a man."

Another lesbian, long experienced with hospital and academic politics, elaborates:

> Men get targeted. In a room full of women with only one man, either the man is focused on, or humiliated and insulted. They don't see lesbians as the same as gay men in nursing. Because a proper nurse is a woman, a feminine woman, a man in nursing already breaks the rules. If the gay man is entrepreneurial and can get along with the old-girls network, then he is less threatening. But I've seen caring gay men be exploited to do unwanted free stuff, while the faculty get all the credit.

A gay academic thinks that the old-girls network favors lesbians and works against gay men. "There's no limit to how high a lesbian can rise, but it would impact how out she can be. Lesbians are more likely to have high positions than do gay men."

A lesbian agrees, "As a female-dominated profession, nursing is a place for lesbians to succeed. Lesbians, regardless of profession, tend to rise to the top because they make work a higher priority and don't have to hunt for husbands on the job."

EFFEMINATE MEN, MASCULINE WOMEN

Everyone agrees that people who fit certain gay and lesbian stereotypes suffer more discrimination. A supervisor says, "If you're mainstream and quiet about it, there's no limit. But effeminate men or masculine women will have problems. There is a vice president who is gay, and the rumor is that he won't be promoted further until he gets married."

The most often cited examples involve effeminate gay men. A lesbian executive says, "Because of the increased potential risk of AIDS, effeminate men are denied consideration for executive positions in hospitals." A gay man says, "I know a very effeminate gay man who was turned down for a director of nursing position for no good reason other than he is an effeminate gay man."

For some, the lavender ceiling is low. A lesbian staff nurse describes how a coworker was prevented from climbing the clinical ladder. "A very savvy, very bright gay nurse in ICU is somewhat effeminate. I have seen him over and over again be denied seats on committees and special projects. Everyone refers to him as Roberta. They are holding back a star."

A GENERATION GAP?

Nurses of different ages seem to hold different opinions about whether being lesbian or gay will limit their success. Young nurses frequently report that sexual orientation does not make a difference. A 22-year-old new graduate emphatically denies that being gay will limit his possible success, "I know it won't stop me." A 27-year-old man agrees, "I'm pretty naive, and I don't know what it's like in corporate America, but I think I'll be recognized for my clinical skills." A lesbian who just graduated from a nurse practitioner program says, "I'm looking to write my own ticket. Because I'm a lesbian, I have a lot of opportunity. I have job security. It's going to happen for me."

Nurses in the middle of their careers are more likely to say they can succeed, as long as they are quietly out and do not offend anyone. "I don't care if you're gay, just act straight. You have to walk the walk, and talk the talk to be promoted."

Women in the middle of their careers were more apt to report that being a lesbian eliminates the career-draining aspects of a traditional heterosexual marriage that subordinates the wife to her husband. A 49-year-old lesbian says, "It's helpful because I don't have a husband to take care of."

A nursing administrator with a long career describes the work environment that shaped lesbians who are now at the peak of their career:

> I would not have been able to survive as an out lesbian. I could not acknowledge my relationships with women as anything else than friends. I always socialized with an entirely different set of gay and lesbian friends away from work. It would have been professional suicide to come out in a community hospital or at a university. I take my career very seriously, and my private life is set to the back and not given much interest or emphasis. You don't share your life with your lover in the same way that a heterosexual would share with his spouse. Obviously, my lover could not accompany me to hospital functions. I resented that.

Surprisingly, some of the most out nurses interviewed for this book were also the oldest nurses. Unfortunately, few nurses volunteered to be interviewed who are older than 55 years. The experiences of retired lesbian and gay nurses are a rich resource still waiting to be tapped.

PRACTICE SETTING

It is hard to find a kind of practice setting that is lesbian- and gay-friendly. Some nurses warn of coming out at a Catholic hospital, and others extend that warning to any employer with a religious affiliation. Others see a difference between hospitals and community agencies. An experienced nurse says, "Community nurses are more tolerant, hospital nurses are more controlling."

AIDS units and community agencies have provided many career opportunities for gay and lesbian nurses. But a woman says, "Lesbians and gays would succeed regardless of what we do. Maybe there's a little more permission in AIDS work than in other areas. But if there wasn't AIDS, we would have done something else that we would have been out in."

ACADEMIA

Every nursing instructor interviewed for this book agrees that schools of nursing do not promote openly gay and lesbian nurses. Universities are as bad or worse than community colleges. An instructor says:

> Lesbians are good workers, their careers are important. They do the lion's share of the work in the university, a lot of unsung work. But there's all this resistance to a lesbian getting tenure, but it won't be put on the table. Lesbians can be department heads, but never deans. In some schools, deans are under the scrutiny of the religious right, and gays and lesbians are really just a liability.

Another professor explains, "The dean position was open, and my name was mentioned. But a high-level faculty member warned me that people might think I was a lesbian. I asked if she thought that might be the deciding factor. Yes, she answered, if it was found out. The current dean was quoted as saying we don't have that element here. Little did she know how many she had hired."

In another example, an interview for a deanship came to an abrupt halt when the candidate mentioned her partner. The position was "no longer available."

A lesbian professor describes a similar experience, "A colleague, a brilliant woman and prolific writer, was turned down for an assistant dean position because she's gay. Nothing goes unscrutinized, even your family life. I'll never apply to be a dean for that reason. I'm more comfortable being a faculty member, and helping the people I can."

Sometimes discrimination hides behind polite language. A lesbian insider knows of an administrator who said, "I will not consider a dean candidate who is unmarried or has never been married."

One instructor always comes out during interviews because she values being an out role model for students. The results are frequently bad. "One woman called back to say that she couldn't offer me a job, but that she admired me for wanting to work as an out lesbian."

The closet community scrutinizes the moves of other gay and lesbian instructors. An out instructor says, "Everybody knows your business, and there's a tremendous rumor mill. Every place I interviewed there were closeted lesbians, and they told me about what was being said behind my back. They wanted things changed by someone like me, so that it would change for them."

The situation does not seem hopeful in academia, yet many lesbian and gay faculty members retain their courage. A professor of many years says, "Looking back, I realize that I didn't have to hide so much or compromise so much. The situation nationwide requires more of us to step forward. Many of us are on faculty, some of the best of us."

INTERVIEW OUT?

Many gay and lesbian nurses question whether they should disclose their sexual orientation during an employment interview. A lesbian who is a director at a metropolitan medical center says, "If you're going to be in a highly visible or supervisory position, you should reveal your sexual orientation. It's better to know in the hiring process that you're gay, and that it's a safe place to work."

A lesbian who interviewed for assistant director positions says, "I told the recruiter and the director when I interviewed that I was a lesbian. They told me to keep it quiet. The director almost fell out. She told me that I didn't look like a lesbian. When I asked what a lesbian looked like, she didn't know." She was offered the job, but did not come out to the nurses on the unit.

Diane decided to come out during interviews because she had once lost a job because she is a lesbian. She remembers:

> A woman who wanted to be a vice president and thought that I was a competitor said that I made a pass at her. I lost my job. They fought my unemployment claim, and I had to hire a lawyer. But I won the hearing. I was hurt and angry. I felt betrayed. You want to be honest, and you're honest. Then the people who say it doesn't matter turn around and screw you. So you get gun-shy about telling any straight person. From that point on, I said I was gay in interviews. I'd say, "By the way, I'm a lesbian, does that present any problems?" They would control their faces. They'd tell me they'd

get back to me, then never call. The person who ultimately hired me was a nurse who probably knew gay and lesbian nurses. She didn't give a hoot and a hangnail what you did in your private life.

An academic says, "It depends on whether you want the job or not. It would end the anxiety of whether people would accept you as a dean, because you wouldn't get the job."

Discrimination Is Hidden

Sophisticated employers disguise the lavender ceiling by hiding the real issues. The uncertainty can damage a candidate's confidence and self-esteem. A lesbian who was denied a promotion to a vice-president level recalls:

> I'm not convinced that I didn't get the job because I'm a lesbian. I was relatively well-known as a lesbian. I was an internal candidate, and the top choice of the search committee. There's no way to really know. It felt awful. I had so much internal support. My paranoia gets in the way. Maybe we present ourselves differently. By not presenting all of ourselves, we don't interview well. I don't know.

THE CLOSET COMMUNITY

Nurses in the closet community deny under all circumstances that they are lesbian or gay, and they often go to extremes to appear heterosexual. An experienced academic explains:

> The closet community is very strong and well-connected. Old-time closeted lesbians are reluctant to come out. There's a lot of myths about people who take risks coming out and pay dearly. These myths justify not coming out. I've known women who regularly send themselves flowers with cards signed 'Love, John.' In reality, everybody knows except the lesbian.

An executive in a conservative community hospital describes how staff nurses and administrators alike respected the closet in the past. "Lesbian nurses would deeply closet them-selves so that I would never be forced to discipline them for lesbian issues."

Another nurse agrees, "They're so guarded, and have no spontaneity. It's embarrassing that they're so foolish about who they think doesn't know."

An educator explains:

> There have always been a lot of lesbians in nursing, but closeted lesbians. There's a rift between out and closeted lesbians. It's not an age issue. I've met out older lesbians, and closeted younger lesbians. It involves such powerfully held emotions. There's a big difference between their per-ception and how it really is. It's like a family secret: It's a secret; everybody knows; it's just not talked about.

An out psychiatric nurse has compassion for closeted nurses and their struggle. She explains, "People desperately want a sense of control, and they perceive that the world wants to kill them. So they try to regain control by blaming themselves. I try not to blame closeted people because they're fighting for their lives. It's much bigger than their behavior. They perceive that they live in a hostile environment."

The issues are revealed in a story that may be true or may be an urban legend: Two lesbian lovers worked at the same hospital and kept their long-term relationship very much a secret. They were both near retirement, when one of them had a MI, and the other was on the code team. She performed CPR on her lover, while the whole hospital watched her not respond emotionally to the imminent death of the only person she ever loved.

Do you pity the lovers for the price they paid to remain in the closet? Or hate the hospital for creating the dilemma? Or respect their coworkers for honoring their secret? Or vow to never let it happen to you?

Horizontal Violence

Out lesbian and gay nurses frequently assume that other gay and lesbian nurses are allies, even if they choose to remain closeted.

But fear of exposure can compel closeted people to act in unpredictable and harmful ways. A psychiatric nurse says, "It's painful to think that one of your own kind would hold you back. We do the best we can as a closeted community. It's oppression behavior. We're a people with secrets, and people with secrets are difficult to work with. Many people around us know our secrets, and out of respect for us, keep our secrets for us."

One man told of a gay colleague who as a vice president for nursing in a conservative medical center hospital refused to help a gay staff nurse. The staff nurse recognized that he had a problem with substance abuse and requested a leave of absence without pay to participate in treatment at the Pride Institute, a facility specializing in care for lesbians and gay men. Even though the VP had recently approved a similar leave for a heterosexual female nurse who wanted substance abuse treatment locally, he refused to grant the leave to the gay nurse. "He was afraid that he'd be accused of giving favors to gay people," explains his colleague. "And he was deathly afraid of coming out. Because the Pride Institute was part of the picture, it would raise too many questions that he was unwilling to answer. The most powerful weapon of oppression is self-oppression. Bigots don't have to beat us up, we beat ourselves up for them."

The complexity of horizontal violence also confuses heterosexual allies. An out academic says, "A lot of straight women just don't get it. They don't understand the dynamics of internalized homophobia or horizontal violence; why another gay person is not on your side."

Sometimes feeling a sense of community with other gay and lesbian colleagues creates a dilemma. How do you support peers when their behavior does not warrant support? A director explains, "I didn't want to be the one to betray a lesbian colleague. If it had been anyone else, I would have done something sooner. I wanted lesbians to look OK. I didn't want to fuel people saying, 'Look these lesbians can't have grown-up relationships.'"

Even staff nurses feel a lack of support from other gay and lesbian nurses. A nurse in the Midwest says, "There's a wall between me and the other lesbian nurses. I feel like I'm doing something wrong. Just because we share a sexual orientation, we don't share anything else."

THE COST OF BIGOTRY

As a profession, nursing pays a tremendous price for bigotry. Nurses who directly experience discrimination pay an obvious emotional penalty. But their employers also pay to recruit and train their replacements after a gay or lesbian nurse quits in frustration. Qualified nurses who are denied promotions lose a step in their career, but their employers lose the unrealized rewards of hiring the best candidate.

Witch-hunts, whether in the military, academia, or hospitals, are expensive to conduct and the people ousted are expensive to replace. In the military alone, the General Accounting Office estimates that the training cost from 1980 to 1991 to replace gay and lesbian servicemembers discharged because of their sexual orientation reached $494 million. The actual investigation costs in 1990 alone topped $2.5 million (Cammermeyer, 1994).

Heterosexual nurses also pay a high price because of homophobia. A staff nurse concludes, "Homophobia is a way to limit and threaten us, and it's frustrating that heterosexuals don't recognize that homophobia also limits them."

A professor agrees, "We must expose homophobia for what it is—a hammer to intimidate strong women by labeling them as lesbians. There is all this heterosexual imagery in nursing, and lesbians are punished."

Rather than risking being labeled a lesbian, capable women will accept unjust assignments, working conditions, and compensation. This harms all women and prevents organizing because everyone will be tarred with the same brush of being labeled a lesbian. Rather than risk the label, many women remain isolated.

She further elaborates on the connection between feminism and homophobia:

> Being labeled a feminist is as bad as or worse than being a lesbian. Even demanding equal pay labels you as a feminist. When you look below the surface, nurses are serving the patriarchal system by playing the role of the strong wife. They buckle under the slightest stress, and some serve as token torturers. Self-hatred as a woman is turned outward and expressed in statements such as "nurses eat their young."

Bigotry and the self-hatred that it engenders are also weapons against gay men. According to a gay man who has long served in nursing organizations, "The true weapon of oppression is that other people don't have to beat you up, because you beat yourself harder for being gay."

An insider comments,

> In nursing, we try to save everyone's face, rather than play with a stick. Nurses are on the fringes of where decisions are being made, trying to make themselves acceptable. Nurses don't act, but react to the most powerful people, be they legislators or doctors. Outsiders divide and conquer. And gay and lesbian issues are just another lever, but not openly discussed.

A staff nurse comments on the rigidity of many nurses, "The feminist aspect of their mentality is missing. I'm surprised at their naivete. These are women who have wanted to be nurses since they were little girls. They want orderliness and a hierarchy that defines their place. They're comfortable complaining in a coffee-klatch fashion about doctors behind their backs, but they are afraid to take the real power."

Many non-gay men in nursing are also marginalized by stereotypes. However, non-gay men seldom help to end discrimination for their gay colleagues. Instead, they waste time and energy convincing others that they are not gay. Or they shun gay men to avoid guilt by association. A lesbian executive says, "Straight men are so afraid of being perceived as gay, that they don't even associate with each other."

SUCCESSFUL GAY AND LESBIAN MANAGERS

A handful of middle managers and instructors report being openly out at work and receiving support from their employers. They follow a middle path between activism and the closet.

Many were well known by the people who hired them. A nurse manager explains, "My decision to be out was strongly influenced by a former openly gay director. She was very positive, and threw it in people's faces almost to the point of activism. Her being out made it easier for me to be out. It's not a shock to be gay here." Another says, "I didn't have to break ground here. No one seemed scared or nervous about lesbians."

Their supervisors value honesty or personal authenticity. A nurse manager says, "My bosses admire me more for being honest. In their eyes, I must not have anything to hide, if I don't hide being gay." They are nonconfrontational about non-work-related lesbian and gay issues, and they are easy to get along with by nature.

Although they have worked for the same hospital for a number of years, they admit that they could easily change jobs if the political climate became discriminatory. Says one, "I wouldn't be afraid to make a career change because of their ignorance."

They offer their expertise as lesbian and gay people to help with patient care. A nurse manager says, "There have been gay patients. The staff was uncomfortable, and they used me as a role model. After watching me, they could care for the patient with relative ease."

They have an egalitarian style of management in terms of sexual orientation, and they move beyond rhetoric to examine the individual. Says one, "I think that you can be a jerk and it can have nothing to do with whether you are gay. The way that people treat you may have less to do with homophobia and more to do with being a jerk." On the other hand, they are quick to step in to stop derogatory remarks or conflicts based on sexual orientation.

A UNIQUE GAY AND LESBIAN CONTRIBUTION

Across all practice specialties, nurses report a unique perspective that they bring to nursing as lesbians and gay men. They describe an open-minded, patient-centered approach that comes from knowing discrimination firsthand. A lesbian explains, "It may have helped me personally to look at my patients from outside my own fishbowl view and see that patients have their own motivations. I believe I have a more empathetic view toward people who are persecuted, such as IV drug users. A straight nurse might deny them pain medication post-op, when it has no relevance to the current situation."

Some nurses are proud that as gay men and lesbians they do not participate in the usual sexual politics. A gay man says, "Minorities and women feel less threatened by gay male nurses because we come across without sexual intent. Other nurses feel less threatened because I'm gay, that they can talk more freely."

Another man describes gay men as practicing outside the confining gender stereotypes that shackle non-gay men. "Straight men in nursing are afraid to touch patients in a comforting way. So being gay enables me to break the barrier."

Many out nurses also serve as experts on lesbian and gay issues. "We can act as resources to people who have questions about gay people." Another says, "People tell me that they answer their children's questions differently now that they know me as a lesbian. One coworker said that her daughter asked her if two women can get married. Her husband said no, but she said yes, and admitted that her answer would have been different two years ago, before she met me."

Maturity is the most valuable quality that out gay and lesbian nurses bring to their practice. "People who are out can function with a greater sense of integrity," says an experienced nurse. "They have more energy by not dividing themselves. They've faced the challenge of coming out and take greater risks."

SUMMARY

For too many lesbian and gay nurses, the lavender ceiling prevents them from fully contributing to their profession while acknowledging all of the diverse parts of their lives. The calculus of the exact height of the ceiling is complicated by the interacting dynamics of age, gender, practice setting, and fear. Whether the ceiling is erected by others out of ignorance and bigotry, or self-imposed out of fear of disclosing sexual orientation, the result is the same—their careers and their contribution to nursing are undermined. When they leave because of discrimination or frustration, they are expensive to replace. Discrimination also victimizes the employer and the patient.

The lavender ceiling hurts all nurses including hetero-sexuals. Masculine or strong women and effeminate men may be discriminated against directly. For all nurses, the potential power of our profession is diminished when women and men are pitted against each other, when closeted nurses fear those who are out, and when labeling someone gay or lesbian is used as a weapon instead of a fact. The health and strength of nursing depends on celebrating and nurturing the rich diversity of all nurses, including the largest minority group—lesbian and gay nurses.

References

Cammermeyer, M. (1994). *Serving in silence.* New York: Viking.

CITY OF ANN ARBOR, MICHIGAN—DOMESTIC PARTNERSHIP INFORMATION SHEET

The Ann Arbor City Council approved the Domestic Partnership Ordinance on November 4, 1991, and in doing so announced the following purposes:

Many persons today share a life as families in enduring and committed relationships apart from marriage. Some are lesbians, some are gay males, some are bisexual persons, and some are heterosexual persons. The City of Ann Arbor has an interest in strengthening and supporting all caring, committed and responsible family forms. The City has also long recognized the importance of cultural diversity and equal treatment and, toward that end, has adopted a human rights ordinance which protects its citizens from discrimination based on, among other things, marital status and sexual orientation.

This domestic partnership ordinance furthers the City of Ann Arbor's interest in families and in cultural diversity and equal treatment by establishing a mechanism for the public expression, sanction, and documentation of the commitment reflected by the domestic partnership, whose members cannot legally marry or choose not to marry. It provides appropriate public recognition of these relationships.

The purpose of this sheet is to provide some additional information about Domestic Partnerships. You need to know that:

There Are Two Ways to Enter a Partnership

The first way is to fill in the Declaration of Domestic Partnership, have it notarized by a notary public and signed by two witnesses, file it with the City Clerk, and pay a fee of $20 if you are a resident (or $25 if you are a nonresident). After three working days, the Clerk will then issue you a Certificate of Domestic Partnership. The Declaration on file with the Clerk then becomes a public document available for others to see.

The second way to enter a partnership is to fill in the Declaration, have it notarized and witnessed, and then retain copies for yourselves. Under this approach, you would not file the Declaration with the Clerk and would not receive the Certificate of Domestic Partnership. No public record of your partnership would exist.

The Domestic Partnership Statement Must Be Notarized

You will each need to sign the domestic partnership statement in front of a notary public and in the presence of two witnesses. You and your partner may wish to sign at the same time but you do not have to do so. If you wish, a different notary may be used for each of you.

Registering Creates No Rights or Benefits

Executing a Declaration of Domestic Partnership will NOT give you (or your partner) the right to any benefits or impose on you (or your partner) any legal responsibilities.

You Still Need a Will

If you desire your partner to get your property when you die, you need a will or some other estate planning tool such as a trust. The Michigan legislature has recognized a standard will form that people can use if they wish. Additionally, Michigan law allows for handwritten wills if they are signed and witnessed. It is best to get legal advice in drafting a will, but statutory wills and other form wills are available at office supply stores.

You Should Consider Executing a Patient Advocate Form and a Power of Attorney for Financial Matters

The only way to be certain that your partner can make decisions about your care if you become too incapacitated to make decisions for yourself is to execute a Patient Advocate form. The only way to make certain that your partner can make decisions or take actions for you about financial matters, if you become too incapacitated to make decisions or take such actions yourself, is for you to execute a financial Power of Attorney. (For a copy of a Patient Advocate form and an explanatory booklet, send $2.00 to Patient Advocate, Michigan State Medical Society, P.O. Box 950, East Lansing, MI, 48826-0950. You may also wish to consult with an attorney. For a power of attorney for financial matters, you should consult with an attorney.)

Registering as Domestic Partners Will Not Create Joint Rights in Property

Entering a domestic partnership has no effect on property ownership. If you and your partner want to buy a home together or a car together, you should check with an attorney about the best way to handle the title.

Ending a Partnership

A domestic partnership ends when: (a) either you or your partner dies or marries; or (b) one or both of you fills out a Termination of Domestic Partnership Form available at the City Clerk's Office or sends the City Clerk a notarized notice saying

that the partnership has ended; or (c) in the case of a partnership for which the Declaration of Domestic Partnership was not
originally filed with the City Clerk, either both sign a notice that
the partnership has ended and have it notarized or one of you
signs such a notice, has it notarized, and mails it to the other
partner.

B

NATIONAL ASSOCIATION OF SOCIAL WORKERS— POLICY STATEMENT: LESBIAN AND GAY ISSUES

The National Association of Social Workers (NASW) recognizes that homosexuality and homosexual cultures have existed throughout history. Homosexuals have been subject to long-standing social condemnation and discrimination. It is the position of NASW that same-gender sexual orientation should be afforded the same respect and rights as opposite-gender sexual orientation. NASW asserts that discrimination and prejudice directed against any group are damaging to the social, emotional, and economic well-being of the affected group and of society as a whole.

NASW believes that nonjudgmental attitudes toward sexual orientation allow social workers to offer optimal support and services to lesbian and gay people. Social workers and the social work profession can support and empower lesbian and gay people through all phases of the coming out process. The profession must also act to eliminate and prevent discriminatory statutes, policies, and actions that diminish the quality of life for lesbians and gay people and that force many to live their lives in the closet. Social workers must encourage development of supportive practice environments for lesbian and gay clients and colleagues (references omitted).

NASW affirms its commitment to work toward full social and legal acceptance and recognition of lesbian and gay people. To this end, NASW shall support legislation, regulation, policies, judicial reviews, political action, changes in social work policy statements and the *NASW Code of Ethics*, and any other means necessary to establish and protect the rights of all people without regard to sexual orientation. Specific activities include, but are not limited to, working for the adoption of policies and legislation to end all forms of discrimination based on homophobia at the federal, state, and local levels; in social institutions; and in the public and private sectors. NASW will work toward the elimination of prejudice, both inside and outside the profession.

To implement this policy, it is recommended that the association direct specific efforts to the following:

Professional and Continuing Education

- ▾ Collaborate with the Council on Social Work Education (CSWE) to ensure that curriculum policy statements include language addressing discrimination against lesbian and gay people and offer a curriculum that includes content on lesbian and gay cultural issues.

- ▾ Work toward implementation of chapter continuing education programs on practice and policy issues relevant to lesbian and gay people and cultures.

- ▾ Develop and sponsor in-service and continuing education programs to train social workers in human sexuality, with a focus on homosexuality and the needs of lesbian and gay communities. This training must address the biopsychological needs of lesbian and gay cultures, legal issues, ethical dilemmas and responsibilities, institutional heterosexism and its impact, effective interventions, and community resources.

- ▾ Work toward recognition of the emergence of families headed by lesbian and gay people and be prepared to address their particular concerns.

- ▾ Increase awareness within the profession of internalized homophobia, oppression, and heterosexism.

- ▾ Support and ensure practitioners' adherence to the *NASW Code of Ethics* with regard to sexual orientation, holding both the individual social worker and the agency accountable for developing and delivering appropriate and nondiscriminatory services.

▼ Strive for full representation and the establishment of means to affirm the presence of lesbian and gay people at all levels of leadership and employment in social work and in NASW.

▼ Collaborate with CSWE, universities, and other professional associations in research projects related to homosexuality, lesbian and gay cultures, and lesbian- and gay-sensitive practice methods that advance social work practice with lesbian and gay people.

Antidiscrimination

▼ Work in coalition with other mental health professions and stakeholders to help enact antidiscrimination legislation at national, state, and local levels.

▼ Seek repeal of, and actively campaign against, any laws allowing discriminatory practices against lesbian and gay people.

▼ Work in coalition with other mental health professions to change policies that exclude lesbians and gay people from military and other forms of government service.

▼ Encourage broadening of affirmative action statements in social agencies, universities, professional associations, and funding organizations to include sexual orientation.

▼ Work toward implementation of antidiscrimination personnel policies that cover lesbian and gay people within the NASW and agencies in which social workers are employed.

▼ Encourage social workers, social work administrators, and social work educators to take action to ensure that the dignity and rights of lesbian and gay employees, clients, and students are upheld and that these rights are codified in agency policies.

Public Awareness

- ▾ Encourage the development of programs to increase public awareness of the discrimination experienced by lesbian and gay people and of the contributions to society made by lesbians and gay people, through collaboration with educational, mental health, and research organizations serving the lesbian and gay community.

- ▾ Develop and provide the public with programs, training, and information that promotes proactive efforts to end the physical and psychological violence aimed at lesbian and gay people.

Health and Mental Health Services

- ▾ Encourage policies in both the public and private sectors that ensure nondiscrimination, that are sensitive to the health and mental health needs of lesbian and gay people, and that promote an understanding of gay and lesbian cultures.

- ▾ Make available comprehensive psychological and social support services for lesbian and gay people and for families headed by lesbian and gay parents that are culturally sensitive and respectful.

- ▾ Work toward increasing awareness and implementation of programs that address the health and mental health needs of gay and lesbian youths, who are at high risk of suicide.

Legal and Political Action

- ▾ Develop and participate in coalitions with other professional associations to lobby for the civil rights of lesbian and gay people to defeat efforts to limit the civil rights of lesbian and gay people and to advocate for increased funding for education, treatment services, and research in lesbian and gay communities.

▾ Work toward implementation of domestic partnership legislation at local, state, and national levels that includes lesbian and gay people.

▾ Encourage adoption of laws that recognize inheritance, insurance, child custody, property, and other rights in lesbian and gay relationships.

▾ Seek election of self-identified lesbian and gay candidates in all political jurisdictions.

▾ Develop and disseminate model antidiscrimination and domestic partnership legislation that can be used in municipal, state, and national legislatures.

(From *Social Work Speaks*, 3rd edition. Reprinted with permission. Copyright 1994 by the National Association of Social Workers, Inc.)

AMERICAN PSYCHOLOGICAL ASSOCIATION COMMITTEE ON LESBIAN AND GAY CONCERNS: AVOIDING HETEROSEXUAL BIAS IN LANGUAGE

Problems of Terminology

Problems occur in language concerning lesbians, gay men, and bisexual persons when the language is too vague or the concepts are poorly defined. There are two major problems of designation. Language may be ambiguous in reference, so that the reader is uncertain about its meaning or its inclusion and exclusion criteria; and the term *homosexuality* has been associated in the past with deviance, mental illness, and criminal behavior, and these negative stereotypes may be perpetuated by biased language.

1. The term *sexual orientation* is preferred to *sexual preference* for psychological writing and refers to sexual and affectional relationships of lesbians, gay, bisexual, and heterosexual people. The word *preference* suggests a degree of voluntary choice that is not necessarily reported by lesbians and gay men and that has not been demonstrated in psychological research.

    The terms *lesbian sexual orientation, heterosexual orientation, gay male sexual orientation,* and *bisexual sexual orientation* are preferable to *lesbianism, heterosexuality, homosexuality,* and *bisexuality.* The former terms focus on people, and some of the latter terms have in the past been associated with pathology.

2. *Lesbian* and *gay male* are preferred to the word *homosexual* when used as an adjective referring to specific persons or groups, and the terms *lesbians* and *gay men* are preferred to *homosexuals* used as nouns when referring to specific persons or groups. The word *homosexual* has several problems of designation. First, it may perpetuate negative stereotypes because of its historical associations with pathology and criminal behavior. Second, it is ambiguous in reference because it is often assumed to refer exclusively to men and thus renders lesbians invisible. Third, it is often unclear.

The terms *gay male* and *lesbian* refer primarily to identities and to the modern culture and communities that have been developed among people who share those identities. They should be distinguished from sexual behavior. Some men and women have sex with others of their own gender but do not consider themselves to be gay or lesbian. In contrast, the terms *heterosexual* and *bisexual* currently are used to describe both identity and behavior.

The terms *gay* and *gay persons* as nouns have been used to refer to both males and females. However, these terms may be ambiguous in reference because readers who are used to the terms *lesbian* and *gay* may assume that *gay* refers to men only. Thus it is preferable to use *gay* or *gay persons* only when prior reference has specified the gender composition of this term.

Terms such as *gay male* are preferable to *homosexuality* or *male homosexuality*, as are grammatical reconstructions (e.g., "his colleagues knew he was gay" rather than "his colleagues knew about his homosexuality"). The same is true for *lesbian* in place of *female homosexual, female homosexuality,* or *lesbianism.*

3. *Same-gender sexual behavior, male-male sexual behavior,* and *female-female sexual behavior* are appropriate terms for specific instances of same-gender sexual behavior that people engage in regardless of their sexual orientation (e.g., a married heterosexual man who

once had a same-gender sexual encounter). Likewise, it is useful that women and men not be considered "opposites" (as in *opposite sex*) to avoid polarization, and that heterosexual women and men not be viewed as opposite to lesbians and gay men. Thus *male-female behavior* is preferred to the term *opposite-sex behavior* when referring to specific instances of other-gender sexual behavior that people engage in regardless of their sexual orientation.

When referring to sexual behavior that cannot be described as heterosexual, gay, lesbian, or bisexual, special care needs to be taken. For example, descriptions of sexual behavior among animal species should be termed *male-male sexual behavior* or *male-female sexual behavior* rather than *homosexual behavior* or *heterosexual behavior.*

4. *Bisexual women and men, bisexual persons,* and *bisexual* as adjectives refer to people who relate sexually and affectionally to women and men. These terms are often omitted in discussions of sexual orientation and thus give the erroneous impression that all people relate exclusively to one gender. Omission of the term *bisexual* also contributes to the invisibility of bisexual women and men. Although it may seem cumbersome at first, it is clearest to use the term *lesbians, gay men,* and *bisexual women or men* when referring inclusively to members of these groups.

5. *Heterosexual* as an adjective is acceptable for people who have male-female affectional and sexual relationships and who do not engage in sexual relationships with people of the same gender.

6. The terms *sex* and *gender* are often used interchangeably. Nevertheless, the term *sex* is often confused with sexual behavior, and this is particularly troublesome when differentiating between sexual orientation and gender. For example, the phrase "it was sexual orientation, rather than gender, that accounted for most of the variance" is clearer than "it was sexual orientation, rather than sex, that accounted for most of the variance." In

the latter phrase, *sex* may be misinterpreted as referring to sexual activity. It is generally more precise to use the term *gender.*

Goals for Reducing Heterosexual Bias in Language

1. *Reducing heterosexual bias and increasing visibility of lesbians, gay men, and bisexual persons.* Lesbians, gay men, and bisexual men and women often feel ignored by the general media, which take the heterosexual orientation of the reader for granted. Unless an author is referring specifically to heterosexual people, writing should be free of heterosexual bias. Ways to increase the visibility of lesbians, gay men, and bisexual persons include the following:

   a. Using examples of lesbians, gay men, and bisexual persons when referring to activities (e.g., parenting, athletic ability) that are erroneously associated only with heterosexual people by many readers.

   b. Referring to lesbians, gay men, and bisexual persons in situations other than sexual relationships. Historically, the term *homosexuality* has connoted sexual activity rather than a general way of relating and living.

   c. Omitting discussion of marital status unless legal marital relationships are the subject of the writing. Marital status per se is not a good indicator of cohabitation (married couples may be separated, unmarried couples may live together), sexual activity, or sexual orientation (a person who is married may be in a gay or lesbian relationship with a partner). Furthermore, describing people as either married or single renders lesbians, gay men, and bisexual persons as well as heterosexual people in cohabitating relationships invisible.

   d. Referring to sexual and intimate emotional partners with both male and female terms (e.g., "the adolescent males were asked about the age at which they first had a male or female sexual partner").

e. Using sexual terminology that is relevant to lesbians and gay men as well as bisexual and heterosexual people (e.g., "when did you first engage in sexual activity" rather than "when did you first have sexual intercourse").

f. Avoiding the assumption that pregnancy may result from sexual activity (e.g., "it is recommended that women attending the clinic who currently are engaging in sexual activity with men be given oral contraceptives," instead of "it is recommended that women who attend the clinic be given oral contraceptives").

2. *Clarity of expression and avoidance of inaccurate stereotypes about lesbians, gay men, and bisexual persons.* Stigmatizing or pathologizing language regarding gay men, lesbians, and bisexual persons should be avoided (e.g., "sexual deviate," "sexual invert"). Authors should take care that examples do not further stigmatize lesbians, gay men, or bisexual persons. An example such as "Psychologists need training in working with special populations such as lesbians, drug abusers, and alcoholics" is stigmatizing in that it lists a status designation (lesbians) with designations of people being treated.

3. *Comparisons of lesbians or gay men with parallel groups.* When comparing a group of gay men or lesbians to others, parallel terms have not always been used. For example, contrasting lesbians with the "general public" or "normal women" portrays lesbians as marginal to society. More appropriate comparison groups might be "heterosexual women," "heterosexual men and women," or "gay men and heterosexual women and men."

Source: Committee on Lesbian and Gay Concerns. (1991). Avoiding heterosexual bias in language. *American Psychologist,* 46(9), 973–974. This reprint omits the article's introduction.

Appendix

D | SUGGESTED READING

American Academy of Nursing Expert Panel on Culturally Competent Nursing Care. (1992). Culturally competent health care. *Nursing Outlook, 40*(6), 277–283.

American Civil Liberties Union. (undated). *Legislative briefing series number 1: Domestic partnerships.* New York: Author.

American Civil Liberties Union. (undated). *The Americans with Disabilities Act: What it means for people living with HIV disease, questions and answers.* New York: Author.

American Nurses Association. (1994). *Nursing and HIV/AIDS.* Washington, DC: American Nurses Publishing.

Bennett, M. J. (1986). A developmental approach to training for inter-cultural sensitivity. *International Journal of Intercultural Relationships, 10,* 179–196.

Blummenfeld, W. J. (Ed.). (1992). *Homophobia: How we all pay the price.* Boston: Beacon.

Bradford, J., Ryan, C., & Rothblum, E. D. (1994). National lesbian health care survey: Implications for mental health care. *Journal of Consulting & Clinical Psychology, 62*(2), 228–242.

Browing, C. (1987). Therapeutic issues and intervention strategies with young adult lesbian clients: A developmental approach. *Journal of Homosexuality,* 14(1–2), 45–52.

Buenting, J. A. (1992). Health life-styles of lesbians and heterosexual women. *Health Care for Women International, 13*(2), 165–171.

Cammermeyer, M. (1994). *Serving in silence.* New York: Viking.

Cass, V. C. (1979). Homosexual identity formation: A theoretical model. *Journal of Homosexuality, 4*(5), 219–235.

Clunis, D. M., & Green, G. D. (1993). *Lesbian couples: Creating healthy relationships for the '90s.* Seattle: Seal.

Cruikshank, M. (1990). Lavender and gray: A brief survey of lesbian and gay aging studies. *Journal of Homosexuality, 20*(3–4), 77–87.

Deevey, S. (1990). Older lesbian women: An invisible minority. *Journal of Gerontological Nursing, 16*(5), 35–39.

Deevey, S. (1993). Lesbian self-disclosure: Strategies for success. *Journal of Psychosocial Nursing, 31*(4), 21–26.

Deevey, S. (1995). Lesbian health care. In C. I. Fogel & N. F. Woods (Eds.), *Women's health care: A comprehensive handbook* (pp. 189–206). Thousand Oaks, CA: Sage.

Deevey, S., & Wall, L. J. (1992). How do lesbian women develop serenity? *Health Care for Women International, 13*(2), 199–208.

Eliason, M. J. (1993). AIDS-related stigma and homophobia: Implications for nursing education. *Nurse Educator, 18*(6), 27–30.

Eliason, M. J. (1993). Cultural diversity in nursing care: The lesbian, gay, or bisexual client. *Journal of Transcultural Nursing, 5*(1), 14–20.

Eliason, M. J., Donelan, C., & Randall, C. (1992). Lesbian stereotypes. *Health Care for Women International, 13*(2), 131–144.

Eliason, M. J., & Randall, C. E. (1991). Lesbian phobia in nursing students. *Western Journal of Nursing Research,* 13(3), 363–374.

Finnegan, D. G., & McNally, E. B. (1987). *Dual identities: Counseling chemically dependent gay men and lesbians.* Center City, MN: Hazelden.

Friend, R. A. (1990). Older lesbian and gay people: A theory of successful aging. *Journal of Homosexuality, 20*(3–4), 99–118.

Garnets, L., Hancock, K. A., Cochran, S. D., Goodchilds, J., & Peplau, L. A. (1991). Issues in psychotherapy with lesbian and gay men: A survey of psychologists. *American Psychologist, 46*(9), 964–972.

Gautier, E. (1993). *The legal rights and obligations of HIV-infected health care workers.* San Francisco: American Association of Physicians for Human Rights and New York: the National Lawyers Guild.

Gentry, S. F. (1992). Care for lesbians in a homophobic society. *Health Care for Women International, 13*(2), 173–180.

Gillow, K. E., & Davis, L. L. (1987). Lesbian stress and coping methods. *Journal of Psychosocial Nursing and Mental Health Services, 25*(9), 28–32.

Gonsiorek, J. C., & Weinrich, J. D. (Eds.). (1991). *Homosexuality: Research implications for public policy.* Newbury Park, CA: Sage.

Gooch, S. (1989). Lesbian health issues. *Nursing Standards, 3*(23), 42.

Harvey, S. M., Carr, C., & Bernheine, S. (1989). Lesbian mothers. Health care experiences. *Journal of Nurse-Midwifery, 34*(3), 115–119.

Henderson, D. J., Sampselle, C., Mayes, F., & Oakley, D. (1992). Toward culturally sensitive research in a multicultural society. *Health Care for Women International, 13*(2), 339–350.

Herdt, G., & Boxer, A. (1993). *Children of Horizons: How gay and lesbian teens are leading a new way out of the closet.* Boston: Beacon.

Hitchcock, J. M., & Wison, H. S. (1992). Personal risking: Lesbian self-disclosure of sexual orientation to professional health care providers. *Nursing Research, 41*(3), 178–183.

Kahn, M. J. (1991). Factors affecting the coming out process for lesbians. *Journal of Homosexuality, 21*(3), 47–70.

Kus, R. J. (Ed.). (1990). *Keys to caring: Assisting your gay and lesbian clients.* Boston: Alyson.

Lambda Legal Defense & Education Fund. (1994). Negotiating for equal employment benefits: A resource packet. New York: Author.

Lucas, V. A. (1992). An investigation of the health care preferences of the lesbian population. *Health Care for Women International, 13*(2), 221–228.

Lynch, M. A. (1993). When the patient is also a lesbian. *AWHONNS Clinical Issues in Perinatal & Women's Health Nursing, 4*(2), 196–202.

Murphy, B. C. (1992). Educating mental health professionals about gay and lesbian issues. *Journal of Homosexuality, 22*(3–4), 229–246.

National Center for Lesbian Rights. (1992). *Recognizing lesbian and gay families: Strategies for obtaining domestic partners benefits.* San Francisco: Author.

Neisen, J. H. (1990). Heterosism: Redefining homophobia for the 1990s. *Journal of Gay and Lesbian Psychotherapy, 1*(3), 21–35.

Neisen, J. H., & Sandall, H. (1990). Alcohol and other drug abuse in a gay/lesbian population: Related to victimization? *Journal of Psychology and Human Sexuality, 3*(1), 151–168.

Pharr, S. (1988). *Homophobia: A Weapon of Sexism.* Little Rock, AK: Chardon Press.

Randall, C. E. (1989). Lesbian phobia among BSN educators: A survey. *Journal of Nursing Education, 28*(7), 302–306.

Remafedi, G. (1990). Fundamental issues in the care of homosexual youth. *Medical Clinics of North America, 74*(5), 1169–1179.

Remafedi, G. (Ed.). (1994). *Death by denial: Studies of suicide in gay and lesbian teenagers.* Boston: Alyson.

Robertson, M. M. (1992). Lesbians as an invisible minority in the health services arena. *Health Care for Women International, 13*(2), 155–163.

Rose, P., & Platzer, H. (1993). Confronting prejudice: Gay and lesbian issues. *Nursing Times, 89*(31), 52–54.

Rubenstein, W. B. (Ed.). (1993). *Lesbians, gay men, and the law.* New York: The New Press.

Sanford, N. D. (1989). Providing sensitive health care to gay and lesbian youth. *Nurse Practitioner, 14*(5), 30–32, 35–36, 39.

Sharkey, L. (1987). Nurses in the closet: Is nursing open and receptive to gay and lesbian nurses? *Imprint, 34*(3), 38–39.

Shernoff, M. (Ed.). (1991). *Counseling chemically dependent people with HIV illness.* New York: Harrington Park Press.

Singer, B. L., & Deschamps, D. (Eds.). (1994). *Gay and lesbian stats: A pocket guide of facts and figures.* New York: The New Press.

Smith, G. B. (1993). Homophobia and attitudes toward gay men and lesbians by psychiatric nurses. *Archives of Psychiatric Nursing, 7*(6), 377–384.

Stephany, T. M. (1988). Lesbian nurse. *Nursing Outlook, 36*(6), 295.

Stephany, T. M. (1989). Lesbian hospice nurse: The visible presence. *American Journal of Hospice Care, 6*(5), 13–14.

Stephany, T. M. (1991). The invisible presence: Gay and lesbian nurses. *California Nursing, 13*(3), 20–21.

Stephany, T. M. (1992). Faculty support for gay and lesbian nursing students. *Nurse Educator, 17*(5), 22–23.

Stephany, T.M. (1992). Promoting mental health: Lesbian nurse support groups. *Journal of Psychosocial Nursing, 30*(2), 35–38.

Stevens, P. E. (1992). Lesbian health care research: A review of the literature from 1970 to 1990. *Health Care for Women International, 13*(2), 91–120.

Stevens, P. E., & Hall, J. M. (1988). Stigma, health beliefs, and experiences with health care in lesbian women. *Image—The Journal of Nursing Scholarship, 20*(2), 69–73.

Thompson, K., & Andrzejewski, J. (1988). *Why can't Sharon Kowalski come home?* San Francisco: Spinster, Aunt Lute Books.

Treadway, L., & Yoakam, J. (1992). Creating a safer school environment for lesbian and gay students. *Journal of School Health, 62*(7), 352–357.

Trippet, S. E. (1994). Lesbians' mental health concerns. *Health Care for Women International, 15*(4), 317–323.

Trippet, S. E., & Bain, J. (1992). Reasons American lesbians fail to seek traditional health care. *Health Care for Women International, 13*(2), 145–153.

Trippet, S. E. & Bain J. (1993). Physical health problems and concerns of lesbians. *Women & Health, 20*(2), 59–70.

White, J., & Levinson, W. (1993). Primary care of lesbian patients. *Journal of General Internal Medicine, 8*(1), 41–47.

Wismont, J. M., & Reame, N. E. (1989). The lesbian childbearing experience: Assessing developmental tasks. *Image—the Journal of Nursing Scholarship, 21*(3), 137–141.

Women's Action Coalition. (Ed.). (1993). *WAC stats: The facts about women.* (rev. ed.). New York: The New Press.

Zera, D. (1992). Coming of age in a heterosexist world: The development of gay and lesbian adolescents. *Adolescence, 27*(8), 849–854.

I N D E X

Note: Page references in **bold** type reference non-text material.

A
Acceptance
  identity, 8–9
    personal needs and, 50
    student nurses and, 141
  relationship stage, 91
Advances in Nursing Science, 177
Affinity groups, 176–179
AIDS
  lost ground due to, 179–180
  number infected by, 102–103
  patients with, 31–32
  supporting research on, 174
Alameda County Nurses Association, Lesbian
    Nurses Interest Group, 176
Alienation, feelings of, 43
American Academy of Nursing, cultural
    competency and, 149
American Nurses Association (ANA)
  code of ethics, 164–167
  position on HIV, 113–114
ANA (American Nurses Association)
  code of ethics, 164–167
  position on HIV, 113–114
ANAC (Association of Nurses in AIDS Care),
    114–115
Association of Nurses in AIDS Care (ANAC),
    114–115

B
Being outed, 46–49
Benefits
  cost of, 97–98
  discrimination and, 85–86

  hospitals offering, 94–95
  organizing, 95–97
  pension, 98
Bereavement leave, 99
Bias, language, avoiding, 172–173
Bigotry
  confronting, 61–62
  cost of, 194–195
  levels of, 12–16
    cultural, 15–16
    institutional, 15
    interpersonal, 13–15
    personal, 12–13
  patients and, 24–25
  reasons for, 16–17
  women and, 25–26
Blending relationship stage, 90
Boss
  lesbians/gays as, 63–64
  see also Coworkers
Bowers v. Hardwick, 78
Building relationship stage, 90

C
California Nurses Association, affinity groups
    and, 176
Cammermeyer, Colonel Margarethe, experience
    of, 70–71
Cassandra, 177–178
Change, constant/unpredictable, dealing with,
    67–68
Chemical dependency, 117–118
  impaired professional programs for, 118–119
  supporting research on, 174

treatment selection, 126–127
  issues concerning, 127–129
Children
  coming out to, 88–89
  custody of, state government and, 76–78
  working with, 34–35
Chinn, Peggy, *Advances in Nursing Science*, 177
Clinics, lesbian/gay, 28–29
Closet community, 191–193
  defined, 5
  working with, 63
Code for Nurses with Interpretive Statements, 164
Collaboration relationship stage, 91
Collective bargaining, benefits and, 96
Coming out, 5–6
  benefits of, 10
  children and, 88–89
  coworkers/managers and, 37–40
    reasons for, 38–39
  forced, 46–49
    dealing with, 47–48
    supportive managers and, 48–49
  methods of, 40–45
  patients and, 23–24
  risks of, 11
  stages of, 6–10
    identify confusion, 6
    identity acceptance, 8–9
    identity comparison, 6–8
    identity pride, 9
    identity synthesis, 9–10
    identity tolerance, 8
    using, 49–50
  student nurses, 134–137
  supporting, 168–169
  see also Outing
Commitment relationship stage, 91
Comparison
  identity, 6–8
    personal needs and, 49
    student nurses and, 140–141
Conflict
  dealing with, 60–62
  relationship stage, defined, 91
Confusion
  identity, 6
    student nurses and, 140
Coping, with stress, 65–66
Coworkers
  coming out to, 37–40

methods of, 40–45
  reasons for, 38–39
discrimination and, 51
  response of, 27–28
supportive, 41–42
unsupportive, 42–43
see also Boss
Cultural
  bigotry, 15–16
  competence, 147–153
    care, 170–173

D
Dating, at work, 64
Discrimination, 50–53
  benefits and, 85–86
  censoring, 166–167
  coworkers, 51
    response to, 27–28
  described, 11
  doctors and, 53
  domestic partner, 87
  ending, 164–169
    ANA code of ethics and, 164–167
    in the military, 166
    national statement, 167–168
    state nurses associations and, 165–166
  faculty and, 146–147
  managers and, 51–53
  patients and, 24–25
  steering as, 32–33
  student nurses and, 145–146
  women and, 25–26
Doctors, discrimination by, 53
Domestic partners
  benefits, 174–175
    hospitals offering, 94–95
  discrimination against, 87
  number of, 87–88
  registering same-sex, 95
  sharing parenting responsibilities, 89
  working with, 65
  see also Partner; Relationships
"Don't ask, don't tell" policy, 59
Drug dependency, 117–118
  impaired professional programs for, 118–119
  supporting research on, 174
  treatment selection, 126–127
    issues concerning, 127–129

E
Effeminate men, 186–187

Employee assistance programs, 175
Employment interview, outing during, 190–191

F
Faculty
    attitudes of, 138–140
    discrimination against, 146–147
    strategies and, 142–144
Fake husbands/wives, military personnel and, 60
Family and Medical Leave Act, 99
Federal government, protection by, 68–69

G
Gay Nurses' Alliance, 178–179
Gays
    affinity groups for, 176–179
    as boss, 63–64
    clinics for, 28–29
    described, 1–2
    estimating number of, 4–5
    growth of relationships of, 90–91
    honoring history of, 169–170
    in the hospital, 29–30
    as managers, 195–196
    as nurses, working with, 62–63
    as parents, 88–89
    as percentage of population, 2–4
        Kinsey report, 3–4
        recent surveys, 4
    relationships of, 92–93
    role models for, 153–155, 184–185
    stereotypes about, 17–18
    unique contributions of, 196–197
Generation gap, 187–188
Gingrich, Judy, advice from, 55–57
Glass ceiling. *See* Lavender ceiling
Government
    federal, protection by, 68–69
    state, protection by, 76–79

H
Hate speech, 146
Health clinics, lesbian/gay, 28–29
HIV
    American Nurses Association (ANA) position on, 113–114
    mandatory testing, 115
    number infected by, 102–103
    nurses infected by, 103
        advice for, 116–117

    legal protection of, 112–113
    profiles of, 103–112
Homophobia
    described, 11
    reactions to lesbian disclosure, **44–45**
Horizontal violence, 192–193
Hospitals
    lesbians/gays in, 29–30
    offering benefits, 94–95
Husbands, fake, military nurses and, 60

I
Identity
    acceptance, 8–9
        personal needs and, 50
        student nurses and, 141
    comparison, 6–8
        personal needs and, 49
        student nurses and, 140–141
    confusion, 6
        personal needs and, 49
        student nurses and, 140
    pride, 9
        personal needs and, 50
        student nurses and, 141–142
    synthesis, 9–10
        personal needs and, 50
        student nurses and, 142
    tolerance, 8
        personal needs and, 49–50
        student nurses and, 141
In the closet, defined, 5
Innes, E. Carolyn, Gay Nurses' Alliance and, 178
Institutional bigotry, 15
Interpersonal bigotry, 13–15

J
Journal of Homosexuality, 173
Journal of Transcultural Nursing, 173

K
Kinsey, Alfred, 3
Kinsey report, homosexuality and, 3–4
Kowalski, Sharon, child custody and, 77–78

L
Labor contracts, 79–81
Lambda Legal Defense and Education Fund, 71
    benefit costs and, 97
Language, avoiding bias, 172–173

Lavender
  ceiling,
    academia and, 189–190
    closet community and, 191–193
    employment interview and, 190–191
    generation gap and, 187–188
    nurses and, 183–184
  network, 185
Legal issues
  boards of nursing, 78–79
  child custody, 76–78
  labor contracts, 79–81
  local government protection, 79
  military and, 69–73
  military personnel, 70–73
    Colonel Margarethe Cammermeyer and,
      70–71
    guidelines for, 72–73
    investigations and, 72
  protection,
    federal government, 68–69
    state government, 76–79
  sodomy laws, 78
  U.S. Supreme Court and, 74–76
Lesbians
  affinity groups for, 176–179
  as boss, 63–64
  clinics for, 28–29
  described, 1–2
  estimating number of, 4–5
  growth of relationships of, 91
  honoring history of, 169–170
  in the hospital, 29–30
  as managers, 195–196
  as nurses, working with, 62–63
  as parents, 88–89
  as percentage of population, 2–4
    Kinsey report, 3–4
    recent surveys, 4
  relationships of, 92–93
  role models for, 153–155, 184–185
  self-disclosure, reactions to, 44–45
  stereotypes about, 18–20
  unique contributions of, 196–197
Levi Strauss & Company, benefit costs and,
    97–98
Local government, protection and, 79

M
Maintaining relationship stage, 90
Managers
  coming out to, 37–40

  methods of, 40–45
  reasons for, 38–39
  discrimination by, 51–53
  supportive, 41–42
    outing and, 48–49
  unsupportive, 42–43
Mandatory testing, HIV and, 115
Masculine women, 186–187
MCC, advice from, 55–57
Men, effeminate, 186–187
Military
  ending discrimination in, 166
  investigations, facing, 72
  legal issues and, 69–73
    Colonel Margarethe Cammermeyer and,
      70–71
  nurses, 57–60
    blackmail of, 57–58
    "don't ask, don't tell," 59
    fake husband, fake wives and, 60
    guidelines for, 72–73
    personal cost of, 59–60
Military Law Task Force, 71
Military personnel, 70–73
  Colonel Margarethe Cammermeyer, 70–71
  guidelines for, 72–73
  investigations and, 72
Montefiore Medical Center, benefit costs and,
    98
Mt. Sinai hospital, bereavement leave and,
    99

N
Nesting relationship stage, 90
New York Nurses Association, bereavement
    leave and, 99
Nurses
  chemically dependent, 117–118
    advice to, 129–130
    impaired professional programs for,
      118–119
    profiles of, 119–126
    treatment selection, 126–129
  diversity among, 149
  HIV infected, 103
    advice for, 116–117
    legal protection of, 112–113
    profiles of, 103–112
  lavender,
    ceiling and, 183–184
    network, 185
  military, 57–60

blackmail of, 57–58
"don't ask, don't tell," 59
fake husband, fake wives and, 60
personal cost of, 59–60
Nursing
schools,
cultural view of, 150–151
finding supportive, 155–157
state boards of, 78–79
students,
clinicals, 144
coming out, 134–137
discrimination against, 145–146
faculty and, 138–144
responsibilities to, 134
student attitudes and, 137–138
supporting, 140–142

O

Outing
dealing with, 47–48
described, 46
forced, 46–49
dealing with, 47–48
supportive managers and, 48–49
see also Coming out
Outsider, feeling like an, 43

P

Parents
gays/lesbians as, 88–89
sharing responsibilities, 89
Partner. *See* Domestic partners
Patients
with AIDS, 31–32
coming out to, 23–24
discrimination by, 24–25
women, 33–34
Peer Support for the HIV-Positive Nurse,
114
Pennsylvania State Nurses Association, Gay
Nurses' Alliance and, 178
Pension benefits, 98
Personal bigotry, 12–13
Placement discrimination, 32–33
Prejudice
levels of, 12–16
cultural, 15–16
institutional, 15
interpersonal, 13–15
personal, 12–13
reasons for, 16–17

sectarian beliefs and, 53–57
advice from MCC concerning, 55–57
Prerelationship stage, 91
Pride
identity, 9
personal needs and, 50
student nurses and, 141–142
Protection
federal government and, 68–69
labor contracts and, 79–81
local government and, 79
military and, 69–73
state government and, 76–79
U.S. Supreme Court and, 74–76

R

Radical Feminist Nurses Newsjournal, 178
Relationships
comparing, 92
gay/lesbian, 92–93
growth of,
gays, 90–91
lesbians, 91
naming committed, 86
sanctions for, 94
see also Domestic partners
Releasing relationship stage, 90
Religious beliefs, sectarian beliefs and, 53–57
Renewing relationship stage, 91
Research, supporting, 174
Role models, 153–155, 184–185
Romance relationship stage, 91

S

Sectarian beliefs, prejudice based on, 53–57
Serving in Silence, 70, 71
Sexes, differences between, 185–186
Significant other, working with, 65
Sodomy laws, state, 78
State boards of nursing, 78–79
State government
protection by, 76–79
sodomy laws and, 78
Steering, described, 32–33
Stereotypes
gays, 17–18
lesbians, 18–20
Stress, dealing with, 65–66
Student nurses
clinicals, 144
coming out, 134–137
discrimination against, 145–146

faculty,
attitudes and, 138–140
strategies and, 142–144
responsibilities to, 134
student attitudes and, 137–138
supporting, 140–142
Supreme Court, legal issues and, 74–76
Synthesis
identity, 9–10
personal needs and, 50
student nurses and, 142

T
Thompson, Karen, child custody and, 77–78
Tolerance
identity, 8
personal needs and, 49–50
student nurses and, 141

U
Unions, influencing benefits without, 96–97

Universal Fellowship of Metropolitan Community Churches (MCC), advice from, 55–57
University of Michigan, benefits and, 94–95
University of Pennsylvania, health system, 95
Unpaid leave, 99

V
Violence, 146
horizontal, 192–193

W
Waldron, David, Gay Nurses' Alliance and, 178
Wives, fake, military nurses and, 60
Women
discrimination and, 25–26
masculine, 186–187
patients, 33–34
Work
dating at, 64
with your partner, 65

Z
Zilly, Judge Thomas, 71